OCCUPATIONAL HEALTH MEDICAL DIRECTIVES AND NURSING PROCEDURES

Douglas W Martin MD

It is recognized and encouraged that occupational health departments may wish to use this book as an official reference tool or as medical directives for an on-site occupational health nursing program. To facilitate this desire, this book includes an agreement page that can be completed by the supervising physician, occupational health nurse, and corporate client representative. Modifications, deletions, and additions to this book for such purposes are allowed, but in no case are duplicative copies of an original book allowed in such circumstances.

This book is independently published using Ingram Spark by
Martin Occupational Medicine, PC
331 West Pinehurst Trail
Dakota Dunes, South Dakota 57049
www.mom-pc.com

First Published Edition: 2022

Previous non-published editions of this work are in existence from 1999-2021 and were made available under direct contractual agreement.

ISBN 9780996124423

The author and publisher of this work have checked with sources believed to be reliable in their efforts to confirm the accuracy and completeness of the information presented herein and that the information is in accordance with the standard practices accepted at the time of publication. However, neither the author nor the publisher nor any party involved in the creation and publication of this work warrant that the information is in every respect accurate and complete, and they are not responsible for any errors or omissions or for any consequences from application of the information in this book

The ideas and opinions provided in this book are intended to provide guidance only and should not be used as a substitute for independent medical judgment and/or examination. It is the responsibility of the health care professional to rely upon their independent experience and knowledge of their patient or individual being evaluated, to determine the best treatment or evaluation course for their patient or individual. The field of medicine and nursing is constantly changing, and the reader should update their knowledge and understanding with current best science. The author and publisher do not assume any responsibility for any loss, injury, and/or damage to cases, persons, or property arising out of or related to any use of the material contained in this book.

FOREWORD

I was first asked to create onsite occupational health nursing protocols in 1996 and embarked upon the endeavor without much direction and certainly with no mentorship. In my research at the time, there seemed to be a hodgepodge of different approaches to the standardization of triage and care provided by nurses in industrial settings; stemming from rigid written rules to the opposite end of the spectrum that simply abided by "standards of care" for any general nurse.

There seemed to be something missing, and given my background in family medicine, I felt that a guidance document that onsite nurses could apply practically and that at the same time could serve as "standing orders" would prove to be useful.

In prior years, I developed an internally used document that served our local hospital system's occupational medicine division. What happened over the years is that I took feedback from many onsite nurses, workers compensation managers, human resource directors, and other colleagues to continuously add to and improve the document.

There are other works that I have seen that could be considered alternatives if not competitors to this guidance document. But the difference is twofold: (1) this is written by an occupational medicine physician with wide ranging experience of 27 years and (2) it is written to be a PRACTICAL guide, not so much oriented to philosophy, academia, or basic science, but more so toward serving as a standard of reference and series of order sets that can be used every day.

At last, some 25 plus years later, I am now getting around to putting this into a published reference manual text. I am doing this only because so many people have asked me to do so. With technology going off into areas that I never thought they would, there are both hard copy and electronic versions available.

ACKNOWLEDGEMENTS

No one ever creates something like this book by themselves and in a vacuum.

Firstly, I wish to thank my family who often put up with my time commitments that I am sure they do not fully understand.

I would also like to thank the many occupational health nurses whom I have had to pleasure of working with while here in the Siouxland area, and the others whom I have had longer distance conversations with about these matters over time. Communication is in itself an artform which contributed mightily to this document.

Lastly, I would like to acknowledge the American College of Occupational & Environmental Medicine and its members, fellows, leaders, and staff. This is an organization that does not get its just due within the larger sphere of organized medicine specialty societies.

AGREEMENT PHILOSOPHY AND ANNUAL REVIEW

The following page contains an example agreement that can be reviewed and signed by the physician medical director who oversees the occupational health nursing program, the on-site occupational health nurse(s) at the facility providing services, and the corporate client representative who is most directly responsible for the coordination of the program (usually, but not limited to, a human resources, workers compensation, or health benefits administrator) if this book is used as a reference or as a medical directive for that facility.

At a minimum, it is recommended that this reference and medical directive be reviewed by all responsible parties at least on an annual basis.

EXAMPLE AGREEMENT

The on-site Occupational Health Nursing Program offers components of service, system, planning, promotion, operation and reporting. The operation component is further subdivided to include first aid and preliminary musculoskeletal conservative care in the workplace setting. The musculoskeletal care component may include treatments beyond what is typical of nursing practice alone and can be considered similar to "standing orders" from the medical director. These "standing orders" are intended to provide an efficient, timely, and low-cost approach to common musculoskeletal conditions.

Each medical director and occupational health nurse should consult their state licensing authorities regarding any scope of practice limitations in this regard and modify such care as necessary.

The Occupational Health Nurses' first responsibilities include *training, maintenance* of injured part, *protocol for movement*, and *evaluation*.

These medical directives are a guideline for the on-site occupational health nurse to assess and evaluate employees in the work setting. They *are not a medical prescription* or a *substitute* for medical evaluation.

The medical directives are to be reviewed annually. It is imperative that the corporation, facility or plant for which the on-site occupational health nurse is assigned understands the scope and purpose of the on-site nurse and the medical directives contained herein. Equally important is the support and understanding of the company and its administration for the program and its goals.

Reviewed and Approved:

______________________________ Date: __________________________

Medical Director

______________________________ Date: __________________________

Occupational Health Nurse

______________________________ Date: __________________________

Company Representative

OCCUPATIONAL HEALTH
MEDICAL DIRECTIVES AND NURSING PROCEDURES

TABLE OF CONTENTS

This page left blank intentionally

Occupational Health Medical Directives and Nursing Procedures

Introduction

These directives are designed to be used by nurses in an occupational health nursing program. These procedures outline the nurses' role in the handling of emergent and non-emergent situations in the occupational health care setting. As is the case with all occupational health "best practices", accurate documentation is of the utmost importance.

There is a plethora of different onsite occupational health nursing services. Not every employer will use every available service. It is also important to note that some employers may have unique needs. It is not the purpose of this document to be all-encompassing or to substitute as a compendium of occupational health practice.

Therefore, there may be times when an employer will request an occupational health nursing service that is not addressed within this guideline. When that occurs, the request should be submitted to the medical director for review. If appropriate, addenda to these guidelines regarding the specific request will be issued and are to be considered an extension of this document.

In every instance, the recommendations contained within these guidelines are based upon evidence-based literature. It should be understood that in some areas, the evidence is weak or does not exist. In these instances, consensus recommendations are provided.

It should be understood that health care is both art and science. Since it is ever-evolving, the recommendations contained within these guidelines may become obsolete or incorrect as new information is published. It is for this reason that these guidelines are to be reviewed at least on an annual basis.

History

Regardless of the injury or illness, a quick and accurate history should be taken to assist in the evaluation of the condition. Components of the history may consist of, but are not limited to the following:

- Symptoms
- Duration or onset of symptoms
- Circumstances of the injury (i.e., where did it occur, how did it occur, who was nearby, etc.)
- History of prior injury
- Aggravating or relieving factors (i.e., what makes pain better or worse)
- Location of symptoms
- Timing of symptoms
- Previous treatment (i.e., what has been done so far)
- Past medical history (i.e., any aggravating medical problems such as diabetes, CHF, bleeding disorders)
- Current medications
- Social history (i.e., smoking, alcohol, recreational and over-the-counter drug usage, etc.)
- Current/regular job.
- How long at current/regular job

Abdominal Injury

Introduction:

Unrecognized abdominal injury remains a distressingly frequent cause of preventable death after trauma. Any patient sustaining significant deceleration injuries, or a penetrating torso wound must be assumed to have an abdominal visceral injury.

There are two types of abdominal injuries – blunt and penetrating. The liver, spleen and kidney are the organs predominantly involved following blunt trauma. The liver, small bowel, colon and stomach are commonly involved in penetrating injuries. As always, history is very important. Critical questions for abdominal trauma include:

A. Time of injury, mechanism and estimated speed of impact for blunt trauma injuries;

B. Time of injury, mechanism of injury and amount of blood at the scene for penetrating wounds.

Treatment:

As for any potentially major injury, resuscitation and management priorities are of key importance.

1. Assess the CAB's (**C**irculation, **A**irway, **B**reathing).
2. Institute Basic Life Support (BLS) algorithm, including AED use, if indicated.
3. Assess circulation with hemorrhage control.
4. Treatment for possible shock (*see shock protocol*).
5. Activate Emergency Medical Services (**911**) system.

6. **DO NOT** remove penetrating objects in the case of penetrating abdominal injuries.

7. Keep patient N.P.O.

8. Communicate to advanced treatment teams at receiving hospital, knowledge and history of incident and injury.

Abrasions

Introduction:

Abrasions are a very common industrial injury. Breaks in the skin are frequently associated with foreign bodies or puncture wounds that can carry dirt and bacteria into the wound.

Treatment:

1. Remove any foreign bodies, if visible.

2. Clean the wound with soap and water (preferred) or Betadine scrub and irrigate with sterile water or saline, if available.

3. Apply clean dressing. May apply topical antibiotic ointment such as Bacitracin, Neomycin, or triple antibiotic ointment. Dressings should be changed at least daily.

4. Inquire as to tetanus prophylaxis status. If tetanus status is not up-to-date, administer Tdap or DT as per the tetanus immunization directive (*see Tetanus Immunization Directive*).

5. See the patient in 2-3 days to reassess and re-dress the wound.

6. Refer to a physician if:

    a. A foreign body is embedded;

    b. The wound appears to be infected (redness, excessive pain, swelling, warmth, purulent drainage);

    c. The wound does not appear to be healing (i.e., no formation of new connective tissue/granulation).

Ammonia Inhalation and Other Respiratory Exposures

Treatment:

1. Remove injured or affected person to fresh air.
2. Monitor airway and cardiopulmonary status via CAB protocol.
3. Give oxygen and CPR if necessary.
4. Activate Emergency Medical Services (**911**) system.
5. Monitor vital signs.
6. Exercise extreme caution in removing victim from an area with a toxic atmosphere. ***It is important to avoid becoming a victim yourself.***

Amputations

Introduction:

Amputation is a catastrophic extremity injury. Patients with amputation injuries require rapid assessment and consultation with a trauma center. Every effort should be made to preserve the severed part in case of partial or complete amputation. Time is of the essence, as an amputated part will remain viable for only 4-6 hours at room temperature, or up to 18 hours if cooled.

Assessment:

I. Objective/Assessment

A. Vital signs: blood pressure, pulse, respiration.
B. Estimated amount of blood loss.
C. Signs of shock.
D. Body part affected.
E. Severity: amount of damage to surrounding tissue; incised or macerated tissue.
F. Degree and type of wound contamination of stump and of severed part (e.g., oil, dirt, chemical, etc.).
G. Neurovascular status – paralysis, pallor.

II. Subjective

A. Determine degree of pain, paresthesia.
B. Determine source of trauma.
C. Obtain a full and accurate history and description of accident if possible. Such information is important to the surgeon for optimum success of treatment.

III. Charting – statement should include:

A. Body part affected.
B. Degree of tissue damage.
   1. Condition of stump.
   2. Condition of severed part.

C. Condition of patient (blood loss, shock, neurological status).
D. Type of wound contaminant.

IV. Treatment

Have other personnel immediately call for ambulance and/or helicopter transportation, based upon your assessment of severity. In general, immediate transport is needed when a major limb is involved and as the injury becomes closer to the proximal end of the extremity. In either case, time is critical, and the occupational health nurse should be prepared in advance with the location of the nearest center and contact numbers for the fastest method of transportation, whether by ambulance or helicopter. Emergency treatment of the digits and smaller parts may be initiated in the occupational medical unit.

A. Nursing care:

1. Airway maintenance. Use CAB protocol.
2. Oxygen as needed.
3. Keep patient NPO.
4. Place patient in supine position. Elevate area or part if possible.
5. Control bleeding with direct pressure. Use tourniquet only as a last resort.
6. Use sterile technique and equipment.

B. Complete Amputation – Stump Care:

1. Control bleeding at amputation site – elevate stump and apply pressure.
2. Place sterile gauze sponges in a sterile basin and saturate with normal saline. (If sterile equipment not available, use cleanest equipment possible.)
3. Place moist sponges over stump, wrap firmly with roller gauze and put water-tight covering (plastic bag) over stump. **DO NOT PUT PLASTIC DIRECTLY OVER STUMP AND DO NOT CLEAN STUMP.**
4. Apply ice pack (avoid dry ice to avoid irreversible damage).

C. Severed Part:

1. Wrap part with moist saline sponges and roller gauze or wrap in towel moistened with saline. NOTE: Keep the severed part as dry as possible and clean. (Keep the saline to a minimum and do not wrap directly in plastic. Keep dressing or towel between severed part and the plastic.) NOTE: Avoid contact between tissue and ice which can cause tissue damage and freezing and prevent re-implantation.
2. Retrieve the severed part no matter what condition it is in and send to hospital with patient.

D. Incomplete (Partial) Amputation:

1. Control bleeding with pressure.
2. Rinse the affected part if possible. Cleansing and irrigation will probably not be feasible as the person will be in pain and questionable shock. Keeping the person stabilized and transferred are the priorities of the nurse.
3. Place partially severed part as close as possible to its anatomical position. Wrap with sterile gauze without constricting already compromised blood flow.
4. Sling and/or support limb.
5. Cover entire limb or digit with a water-tight plastic bag, making sure it is 3 or 4 inches above the injury. Slip a second plastic bag over the first with ice/water, seal with tape.
6. Avoid direct contact between body tissue and ice or ice water.
7. Elevate limb.
8. Tetanus immunization – as per protocol if indicated. Do not delay transportation. Communicate status to accepting medical team.
9. Prepare to transfer to medical center.
10. Document procedure in nurses' notes.

Anaphylactic Shock

Introduction:

Anaphylactic shock develops within minutes or up to one hour following exposure of a susceptible individual to an antigen that is inhaled or injected parenterally, such as an insect sting. An anaphylactic shock should be anticipated with those persons who have a history of allergies. Initial mild symptoms include: edema and itching about the site of injection, apprehension and sneezing. They are followed rapidly by: edema of the face, hands and other body parts; dilation of pupils; rapid and weak pulse; decreased blood pressure and death.

Signs and symptoms occur in various combinations involving mainly four systems;

- Cardiovascular
- Respiratory
- Cutaneous
- Gastrointestinal

Treatment:

Should be instituted rapidly and should include:

1. Maintenance of an adequate airway, including artificial respiratory, if necessary. Use the CAB protocol.

2. Epinephrine is the mainstay of anaphylaxis therapy. **Give epinephrine 1:1000 0.3cc SQ.** May repeat in 5-10 minutes if no contraindications (i.e., cardiac arrhythmias, excessive elevation in blood pressure).

3. Place patient in Trendelenburg position. If there is a visible insect sting, apply a venous tourniquet proximal to the site of the stinger injection, when the sting is on an extremity. Leave it in place until the patient's vital signs are stabilized.

4. Any employee with a severe systemic reaction needs immediate transfer to an emergency facility. All patients treated for an anaphylactic reaction should be seen by a physician.

Asphyxiation

Introduction:

In the case of asphyxiation, it is important to remember the importance of obtaining assistance before removing the employee from the injury site, particularly if this is in an enclosed space. ***It is imperative not to add to the "victim count".***

Treatment:

1. After assistance has been obtained and any appropriate protective measures have been undertaken, remove the employee from exposure while beginning to initiate artificial respiration.

2. Active Emergency Medical Services (**911**) system.

3. Maintain CPR until respiration is restored or until a physician or emergency medical technician orders otherwise.

4. Notify the Medical Director or other physician in charge.

Bite Wounds

Introduction:

Animal, insect or human bites may be a source of potentially severe infection and should be treated with caution even though they may appear benign.

Treatment:

Animal Bites:

1. Wash thoroughly with Betadine solution or soap and water.
2. Irrigate well with sterile saline, if it is an open wound.
3. Apply Betadine ointment or other antibacterial ointment and a clean dressing.
4. Determine tetanus immunization status and proceed as indicated under Tetanus Immunization directive.
5. For animal bites, the incident needs to be reported to the local health department. The health department will assist in determining the need for rabies prophylaxis and for the need of the animal to be kept under observation.
6. Refer all cases of animal bites to a physician if skin has been broken. It is not necessary to send to doctor cases in which skin has not broken or punctured.

Human Bites:

Human bite wounds are notoriously deceptive and are often underestimated and undertreated. While controversies regarding optimal management continue, the basic tenets of meticulous wound care are no different than those for contaminated wounds.

The goals of therapy are to prevent or appropriately treat infection and to minimize the soft tissue deformity. Recognition and early, aggressive treatment are mandatory to prevent infection and associated complications.

Approximately 10-15% of human bite wounds become infected, and this considerable infection rate is multifactorial. Patients often wait until infection is established before presenting late in the course of their injury, thus necessitating medical attention. Wounds evaluated earlier are frequently more extensive than estimated on initial examination by the inexperienced observer and are frequently managed inadequately.

The bacterial inoculum of human bite wounds is rich in oral flora, as saliva contains as many as 100,000,000 organisms per mL, representing as many as 190 different species. Moreover, most of these injuries occur on the hands, and hand wounds of any cause have a higher infection rate than similar wounds in other anatomic locations.

The possibility of transmission of disease through human bites must be considered. Human bites have been shown to transmit hepatitis B, hepatitis C, herpes simplex virus (HSV), syphilis, tuberculosis, actinomycosis, and tetanus. Evidence suggests that it is biologically possible to transmit HIV through human bites, although this is quite unlikely.

In case of human bites, it is not necessary to report to the local health department. Consult with the Medical Director as necessary.

Insect Bites:

1. If history dictates that there is evidence of general allergic reactions, refer for immediate emergency room medical care.
2. If there is no indication of severe allergic restrictions:
   a) Use tweezers/forceps to remove the stinger, if in the wound.
   b) Wash with soap and water (preferred) or Betadine scrub.
   c) Apply cold pack for fifteen minutes.
   d) If indicated, arrange for medical care.
   e) Recheck in one or two days for problems. Refer to a physician for any such concerns.

Bleeding / Hemorrhage

Introduction:

In the case of bleeding associated with a workplace injury, it is important to assess the site of origin for the bleeding. It is also important to assess whether the bleeding may, in fact, be more pronounced than at first appearance. This is important as in early hemorrhagic shock, one does not see hypotension; rather the earliest sign is, in fact, tachycardia. Therefore, since the early signs of hemorrhagic shock may be very subtle, it is important to assess blood loss, in the case of an injury which has produced bleeding.

Treatment:

Mild Bleeding:

Mild bleeding can usually be controlled with simple, conservative measures.

1. The bleeding site should be identified
2. Apply direct pressure with clean gauze until bleeding stops. Refer for suturing if necessary.
3. Cleanse wound with Betadine scrub.
4. Apply clean dressing.
5. Determine tetanus status and administer tetanus prophylaxis, if necessary. (See Tetanus Immunization Directive.)
6. Advise patient of wound care.
7. Follow-up with the patient in 2-3 days during the next clinical session at the client company. Observe for any signs of infection, numbness, tingling, or loss of motion of the affected part; if the injury was on an extremity, refer to a physician should any of these symptoms develop.

Moderate Bleeding:

1. Apply direct pressure with clean gauze until bleeding is stopped.
2. Check vital signs. ***Remember that the earliest signs of hemorrhagic shock are increased heart rate and cutaneous vasoconstriction.***
3. Cleanse with Betadine scrub.
4. Apply clean dressing.
5. Determine tetanus status and administer tetanus prophylaxis, if necessary. (See Tetanus Immunization Directive.)
6. Refer to physician if suture is needed and for any complaints of numbness, tingling, or loss of motion in an extremity.
7. Follow-up at the next clinic visit for signs of infection, numbness, tingling, or loss of motion of the affected part; if the injury was on an extremity, refer to a physician should any of these symptoms develop.
8. If not sent to physician, advise patient of wound care procedures (patient instruction sheet).

Heavy Bleeding:

1. Activate Emergency Medical Services (**911**) system. Have someone from the Company place the call.
2. Assess ABC's.
3. Attempt to establish the bleeding site. If necessary, cut clothing away that may be covering the wound with as little movement as possible. It should be emphasized, however, that the clothing must be removed.
4. Apply direct pressure to the bleeding site with clean gauze. Elevate if no suspected fracture or increase in pain. If direct pressure does not control the bleeding, you may apply pressure to an appropriate pressure point.
5. Notify trauma center receiving patient of situation.
6. Applying tourniquet is third line of control; if necessary, to apply a tourniquet, it should be proximal to site of bleeding and released for 30 seconds every 3-5 minutes.

Blisters

Treatment:

1. Clean with soap and water (preferred) or Betadine scrub.

2. ***Do not*** open blister.

3. Apply clean dressing.

4. If blister is open, apply Betadine ointment or other antibacterial ointment and clean dressing.

5. Seek cause and attempt to correct.

6. Follow-up wound care in 2-3 days.

Burns

Introduction:

Any patient with a burn injury should be treated with a high index of suspicion for the presence of airway compromise, secondary to smoke inhalation. It cannot be stressed strongly enough that a high index of suspicion for the presence of airway compromise must be maintained. It should be noted that care should be taken to avoid burn injuries to the rescuer while attempting to remove the victim from the injury-provoking environment. Signs of airway obstruction may not be immediately obvious. Clinical indications for possible inhalation injury include:

- facial burns
- singeing of the eyebrows and nasal hair
- carbon deposits and inflammatory changes in the mouth and pharynx
- carbonaceous sputum
- history of impaired mentation
- history of confinement in a burning environment

Burns that are encountered in industry may be classified into several different classifications: thermal, chemical, electrical, and radiation (both non-ionizing and ionizing radiation). Sunburns are classified as a subtype of thermal burn. Burns may be classified by depth of injury into partial and full thickness.

General Treatment:

1. Move patient to safe environment.
2. Break contact with causative agent (extinguish flames, flush off liquid chemicals with irritants, brush off powdered chemicals).
3. Airway maintenance with adjunctive equipment.
4. Supplemental oxygen as necessary at high flow rates.
5. Remove constricting jewelry or clothing that is nonadherent.
6. Cover wounds with sterile sheets, keep patient warm. ***DO NOT USE WET DRESSINGS.***

Thermal Burns

First degree burns result in erythema and swelling of the affected area. Pain may be intense, but there is no necrosis or blistering.

Second degree burns affect only the epidermis with some tissue destruction and blistering.

Third degree burns involve complete destruction of the epidermis and necrosis of the hair follicles and sweat glands.

First Degree Burn Treatment:

1. Immerse in cool water or apply cool packs immediately until the burning sensation does not reoccur on exposure to air, for approximately ten minutes.

2. Wash gently with antibacterial soap and water.

3. Apply sterile dressing.

4. May apply topical medication or burn membrane. Bacitracin, Bactroban or Silvadene are acceptable. Recent research into the use of Silvadene indicates that its use delays healing in some circumstances. For this reason, many evidence-based protocols now suggest the use of Aquacel Ag as a preferred first line agent. However, the practicality of stocking Aquacel with the potential for limited use and its cost requires that each situation be evaluated on an individual basis. Any option contained within Table 3, reprinted from the American Family Physician Journal on page 21, is a reasonable option.

5. Recheck in one day.

6. Give patient information regarding wound/burn care.

7. Determine individual's tetanus immunization status.

Partial (Second Degree) and Full Thickness (Third Degree) Burns

It should be noted that with inhalation injury secondary to a thermal burn, pharyngeal thermal injuries may produce marked upper airway edema; and early maintenance of the airway is of key importance. Furthermore, pulmonary manifestations may be subtle and frequently do not appear in the first 24 hours. It is important, therefore, that the patient with a second or third-degree burn be followed up by a physician.

1. Assess the CAB's. Maintain airway. Administer supplemental oxygen if needed.
2. Cool burned area quickly with water. Never apply ice.
3. Do not attempt to break blisters.
4. Do not remove clothing that adheres to burned tissue.
5. *Apply sterile dressing to enclose entire burned area and immediate surrounding skin. Use aseptic technique.
6. Arrange for physician evaluation and/or transportation.
7. Check tetanus immunization status.
8. Follow-up for application of topical medication / burn membrane and dressing changes as per doctor orders.

*Please see topical burn care table for options.

Other areas of concern with thermal burns are:

- Inhalation of the products of incomplete combustion (i.e., carbon particles) and toxic fumes leading to chemical tracheal bronchitis and pneumonia.
- Direct thermal injury producing airway mucosal sloughing and bronchorrhea and pulmonary edema. ***If you suspect an airway injury, activate Emergency Medical Services (911) system to transport patient to the emergency room.***

Table 3. Commonly Used Topical Medications and Wound Membranes

Name	*Type of therapy*	*Characteristics*
Bacitracin	Topical	Narrow antimicrobial coverage; inexpensive; painless; requires frequent dressing changes; can be used on face or near mucous membranes[1]
Mafenide acetate (Sulfamylon)	Topical	Broad-spectrum antimicrobial coverage; penetrates eschar; may delay healing or cause metabolic acidosis; used for deep burns[1,12]
Mupirocin (Bactroban)	Topical	Good gram-positive antimicrobial coverage; expensive; painless; requires frequent dressing changes; can be used on face[1]
SSD (Silvadene)	Topical	Broad-spectrum antimicrobial coverage; painless; requires frequent dressing changes; delays healing; stains tissue; used in deeper partial-thickness burns; relatively contraindicated in pregnant women, newborns, nursing mothers, and patients with glucose-6-phosphate dehydrogenase deficiency or sulfa allergy[1,6,12,24-26]
Aquacel Ag	Absorptive dressing	Silver impregnated; broad-spectrum antimicrobial coverage; decreases dressing changes; reduces pain; decreases use of pain medications; faster wound closure than with standard therapies[12,27]; decreased total cost compared with SSD[33]
Biobrane	Biocomposite dressing	Less pain and shorter time to healing than with SSD; expensive but lower total treatment cost compared with SSD[28-30]; one study showed effectiveness in superficial burns, but high failure rates with mid-dermal depth burns[24]
Hydrocolloids (Duoderm, Urgotul)	Absorptive dressing	Less pain and shorter time to wound closure than with SSD; good for weeping burns; malodorous; opaque[1,31,35]
Impregnated nonadherent gauze (Xeroform, Vaseline gauze)	Nonabsorptive dressing	No antimicrobial activity; messy; provides a nonadherent barrier over the burn for absorptive dressings; used for superficial burns[1]
Silicone (Mepitel)	Nonabsorptive dressing	Expensive; painless; allows seepage of exudates to secondary bandage[1]
Silver-impregnated dressing (Acticoat)	Nonabsorptive dressing	Delivers low concentrations of silver; broad-spectrum antimicrobial coverage; nonadherent; reduces pain; expensive[1,10,12,36]

AFP, Volume 85, Number 1, January 1, 2012, page 30

Chemical Burns (Including Ammonia Burns)

Introduction:

Chemicals that cause burns are usually acids or alkalis. The alkali burns are generally more serious than acid burns, because alkalis penetrate more deeply. Removal of the chemical and immediate attention to wound care is essential.

Treatment:

Chemical burns are influenced by the duration of contact, concentration of the chemical and amount of the agent. Pertinent areas of treatment include:

1. Irrigation with a neutral solution (water) immediately. Flush away the chemical with large amounts of water, using a shower or hose if available, for at least 20-30 minutes. Alkali burns require longer irrigation. If dry powder is still present on the skin, brush it away before irrigation with water. Large scissors should be provided for the rapid removal of clothing soaked with the chemical.
2. Neutralizing agents have no advantage over water irrigation, because a reaction with the neutralizing agent may itself produce heat, damaging the tissue further.
3. Alkali burns to the eye require continuous irrigation during the first eight hours of the burn. Refer to/consult an ophthalmologist.
4. It is important to remove all clothing from involved areas.
5. Refer any chemical burns to a physician for further evaluation.

Electrical Burns

Introduction:

Initial assessment of the electrically burned patient includes:

1. Check the CAB's.
2. Begin CPR, if necessary.
3. Check for signs of shock or respiratory failure and act accordingly.
4. Treat electrical burns as you would thermal burns.
5. Electrical burns should be referred to a physician for further evaluation.

Cardiac Emergencies

Introduction:

Signs and symptoms of possible cardiac disorders may be as follows:

- Pain originating in the chest, behind the sternum, and/or radiating in the left arm, up into the neck or jaw or through into the back. The pain is usually steady and not changed by movement of the body, breathing, breath holding or swallowing. The pain is frequently described as "pressing", "squeezing", or "choking".
- Indigestion.
- Cyanosis or pallor.
- Difficulty in breathing, often aggravated by lying down.
- Palpitations or some indefinable complaint in the chest.
- Weak, rapid or thready pulse.
- Weakness, faintness, pallor, cold or clammy skin, or shock.

Treatment:

Any suspicion of cardiac difficulties should prompt referral to a physician with immediate transportation per ambulance (**911**). Interim care, while awaiting transfer, should include the following:

- Oxygen, preferably by nasal cannula at 5-6 liters per minute (See oxygen section.)
- The CAB's with vital signs.
- Keep the patient lying down, unless breathing becomes difficulty. You may elevate at a 30-degree angle from the waist for patient comfort.

- If able to swallow, give ASA 325 mg to chew while waiting for transport to the ER.

- Should signs of shock or cardiac arrest occur, begin CPR.

Cerebral Vascular Accident (CVA) / Stroke

Introduction:

The possibility of a stroke is a medical emergency, and the patient should be transported to the emergency room as soon as possible. Other disorders may present with symptoms of stroke, but regardless, the patient should be transported emergently.

Treatment:

1. Monitor CAB's.
2. Activate Emergency Medical Services (**911**) system.
3. Monitor vital signs including pupil reaction.
4. Keep patient quiet with head and shoulders elevated.
5. Keep NPO.

Chest Injuries

Introduction:

Contusions or other blunt trauma of the chest, with or without evidence of external injury, may result in injury to the underlying organs.

Treatment:

1. Monitor CAB's.
2. Activate Emergency Medical Services (**911**) system.
3. Monitor vital signs.
4. Control any bleeding, if applicable.
5. Treat for shock (see Shock Directive).
6. Keep patient NPO.
7. Notify emergency room that will receive patient.

Child Abuse (Real or Suspected)

A. If you become aware of a suspected child abuse case told by a co-worker of a suspected abusive parent/guardian:

1. Strongly encourage and assist co-worker to report incident to Department of Human Services.

2. Follow-up with co-worker at next onsite visit.

3. Contact the appropriate state hotline for additional information. All states have child abuse hotlines that are maintained by their respective departments of human or social services. For example:

   - Iowa DHS Child Abuse Hotline 1-800-362-2178
   - Nebraska Child Abuse Hotline 1-800-652-1999
   - South Dakota Department of Social Services 1-800-422-4453

B. If you become aware of a suspected child abuse case told by a suspected abusive parent/guardian:

1. Get as much information as possible.

2. Contact the appropriate Department of Human Services agency to report incident.

3. If you need additional information, contact your local hospital or county health department.

4. You are required by law to report abuse cases in which you have first-hand knowledge (i.e., told to you by a parent).

C. Local hospital or agency child advocacy centers do not replace or duplicate the work of the Department of Human Services (DHS) or law enforcement agencies. To report suspected child abuse contact:

Local Department of Human or Social Services

Phone: ______________________________

Local Law enforcement

Municipal / City Police Department

Phone: ______________________________

County Sheriff's Department

Phone: ______________________________

Additional Resources

____

Phone: ______________________________

____

Phone: ______________________________

____

Phone: ______________________________

Communicable Diseases

For specific information concerning the current state of communicable disease prevention, monitoring, and treatment, a wide variety of resources are available. The single best resource for up to date information can be found at the Center for Disease Control website. This site contains links to a wide variety of communicable disease information resources with easily printable fact sheets that can be distributed to patients. Another excellent resource is the individual State Department of Public Health website. Finally, there are some County Public Health Webpages that have excellent sections that include many downloadable forms and educational handouts.

www.cdc.gov

Example State Website:
www.idph.state.ia.us

Your State Website:

____

Example County Website:
http://www.johnson-county.com/dept_health.aspx?id=4485

Your County Website:

____

Treatment:

1. Prevent exposure to other personnel.

2. Check local health department codes.

3. Refer to private physician for appropriate treatment.

Contusions

Introduction:

Contusions are a very common industrial injury. While they may not be disabling, they are quite painful and may be a significant source of lost productivity. Attention should be paid to the etiology of the injury to determine if it was preventable by changes in equipment or technique or if the injury was due to inattention.

Treatment:

1. Apply ice immediately for 15-20 minutes and every 2-3 hours over the next 48 hours to minimize and relieve swelling. Wrap with non-restrictive ACE bandage.

2. After the initial 48-hour period, apply moist heat for 15-20 minutes, 3-4 times daily.

3. Advise rest and elevation of the affected part, if possible.

4. Advise acetaminophen (Tylenol) 500 mg, two tablets p.o. every 4-6 hours as needed; not to exceed 4000 mg/24 hours. See pharmacy guidelines. May substitute Ibuprofen 200 mg tablets, two tablets p.o. every 8 hours as needed initially, but may increase to four tablets p.o. every 8 hours as needed; not to exceed 2400 mg per day. As a substitute, Aleve (naproxen sodium) 220 mg one to two tablets every 12 hours, or Orudis KT (ketoprofen) 12.5mg one to two tablets every day may be used.

5. If soreness or disability persists longer than 5-7 days, the employee should be referred to a physician.

Hematoma Development

Some soft tissue trauma injuries may develop a hematoma, which is a blood collection typically underneath the skin either within the muscle tissue or in the subcutaneous tissues. Small hematomas may be followed and treated similar to contusions. Moderate to large hematomas should be referred to the physician for possible aspiration. If any hematoma is noted to be increasing in size, referral to a physician is recommended.

Subungual hematomas are blood collections underneath the nail. Subungual hematoma evacuation should only be performed under strict sterile technique usually by the physician, as infection complications are quite common.

Convulsive Disorders (Epileptic Seizures)

Introduction:

Employees known to have a seizure disorder should be required to bring a statement regarding their emergency care from a physician. In compliance with ADA of 1992, refer to Section 6.5 – Confidentiality and Limitations on Use of Medical Information. Medical-related information on an employee must be kept confidential with exceptions regarding:

1. Necessary restrictions on the work or duties of an employee; and

2. If a disability might require emergency treatment or specific procedures.

This should be handled in a confidential manner to protect the employee's privacy. The employee should be encouraged to explain to his family and co-workers what to do if a convulsion occurs.

Treatment:

Emergency care consists primarily of the following:

1. Protect the employee from self-injury.

2. Maintain an unobstructed airway following the seizure. The patient should be turned to a prone or semi-prone position. The head should be turned to the side to allow for drainage of saliva and vomitus.

3. Provide oxygen if necessary.

4. Once the seizure has ended, or in the case of continued seizures, the patient's personal physician should be notified for further instructions. If seizure activity lasts longer than ten minutes or is immediately repeated, arrange transfer for physician evaluation.

Dermatitis

Introduction:

Most cases of dermatitis lasting longer than 5-7 days will probably need to be evaluated by a physician. Considerable help can be gained by a careful history. A careful history will also help determine if the problem is related to work or a personal condition. The history should attempt to ascertain any recent changes in the patient's job prior to the onset of the dermatitis, or any skin exposures to chemical substances in the workplace, such as solvents, chemicals or samples of any such material that might possibly be responsible for the patient's dermatitis. Read these materials carefully and send them along with the patient to the physician. Any data regarding chemical composition of the material (such as would be obtained from a Safety Data Sheet (SDS) sheet) should be sent along. These materials should be sent in the same concentration and form as when the employee contacts it.

Treatment:

Actions that should be taken with the employee with dermatitis include:

For Mild Inflammation:

1. May apply a 0.5% to 1% hydrocortisone cream to the affected area twice daily until clear or referred to a physician.

2. Attempt to ascertain the underlying cause for the dermatitis.

3. Encourage good skin care practices to employee, such as:

    - Avoid hot water.
    - Good hygiene at work, wash during breaks and before going home.
    - Avoid harsh soaps/cleaners.
    - Use barrier product (if available) while exposed to irritants.
    - Use a good skin moisturizer, especially during winter months.
    - Use of gloves if appropriate for protection.

4. If a rash is weeping, the patient should be referred to a physician.

5. Any signs of infection, such as redness, purulent drainage, warmth, drainage, or spreading of affected areas, should be referred to a physician for further treatment.

For Moderate/Severe Inflammation:

a. Refer to physician.

Kerodex 71 or Skin Pro-Tec for Wet Work:

1. Purpose: For the prevention of skin disorders.

2. Policy:

    - Kerodex 71 or Skin Pro-Tec will be utilized by individuals working with irritants with potential for causing skin disorders
    - Contraindications: Kerodex 71 or Skin Pro-Tec will not be applied in the event the individual presents with impaired skin integrity.

3. Procedure: HOW TO APPLY KERODEX 71 OR SKIN PRO-TEC

    a. Wash hands clean and DRY THOROUGHLY.
    b. Squeeze about ½ inch of cream into palm of one hand.
    c. Spread lightly and evenly, rubbing hands together until dry or until cream disappears into the skin.
    d. Apply a second coating in the same manner.

    MAKE SURE THE CREAM IS APPLIED AROUND THE WRISTS, BETWEEN THE FINGERS, INTO THE CUTICLE, AND UNDER THE NAILS.

    AFTER APPLYING THE KERODEX 71 OR SKIN PRO-TEC, hold hands under the cold running water to "set" cream. Dry in the usual manner.

During the next 3-4 hours, the hands may be washed as often as necessary.

If protection is needed for more than 3-4 hours, wash and dry thoroughly and reapply cream as directed above.

When work is finished, wash with mild soap and warm water. (If the work involves contact with highly irritating substances, or when the hands are subject to friction, the cream should be reapplied every two hours.)

Diabetes mellitus

Introduction:

Although known diabetics may seek assistance from the Health Unit in following their physicians' orders, it is more likely they will go to the unit for problems such as:

Insulin Reaction:

Signs and symptoms: Headache, irritability, hunger, cold damp skin, nervousness, blurred vision, rapid heart rate, pallor.

Treatment:

1. Determine last time and dosage of insulin.
2. Give orange juice or other type of sugar replacement.
3. Refer to personal physician.

Impending Diabetic Coma:

Signs and symptoms: Sugar in urine, extreme thirst, urinary frequency, later followed by extreme weakness, dry flushed skin, drowsiness to unconsciousness, tachypnea, peculiar odor to breath (acetone smell).

Treatment:

1. Arrange for transfer to medical facility.
2. Take history.
3. Monitor vital signs.

4. For severe hypoglycemic reaction, glucagon may be administered per the glucagon protocol:

Glucagon, like insulin, is a hormone made in the pancreas. It acts on the liver by converting glycogen to glucose. Products such as Glucagon or Glucagen are safe to use and relatively free of adverse reactions except for nausea and vomiting. Both are usually well tolerated with no cases of human overdosage being reported.

Glucagon and Glucagen are available in a package with supplies needed for administration. These are called a Glucagon Emergency Kit and Glucogen HypoKit and can only be obtained via prescription or authorization in most jurisdictions. It is the responsibility of the diabetic patient, or in the case of a minor their parent or guardian, to provide the original or any replacement of the kit to emergency glucagon providers.

Each Glucagon Emergency Kit or Glucogen HypoKit contains:

- A bottle of glucagon in powdered form.
- A syringe filled with special diluting fluid

Injectable glucagon is also available in a pre-dosed syringe, such as the Gvoke Autoinjector. These autoinjectors typically are available in pediatric and adult dosages, with the adult dosage usually containing 1 mg.

Additionally, glucagon is now available via nasal powder spray with a trade name Baqsimi. This is a single dose unit that contains 3 mg.

Storage:

Vials of glucagon as well as the diluting solution should be stored at room temperature (59 – 86 F). The powder should not be mixed with the diluting solution until just before it is injected during a hypoglycemic emergency. Glucagon can be given as an injection in accordance with the manufacturer instructions. The injection should be done in the loose, fatty tissue or muscle of the arm or thigh and any unused portion should be discarded. The glucagon solution should not be used unless it is clear and has a water-like consistency. The glucagon emergency provider is advised to check expiration dates on the glucagon emergency kits periodically.

Access:

In addition, plans should be in place to assure the glucagon emergency kits are readily available and in close proximity of the person with diabetes. Consideration of transportation activities such as off facility functions must be considered when planning emergency measures for possible hypoglycemia of the diabetic patient. Depending upon the age of the patient, it may be advisable for them to carry their own glucagon emergency kits during these special activities, and proper documentation of this with review by the glucagon emergency providers is necessary.

Dosage:

In most cases, injectable glucagon is given at a 1 mg dosage for adults and 0.5 mg for children who weigh less than 20 kg (44 pounds). Typically, the recommendations state that a second dose may be administered pending emergency medical transport if the patient does not respond to the first dose.

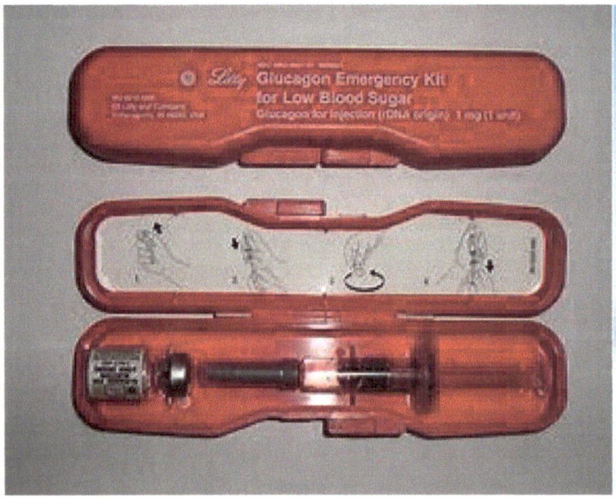

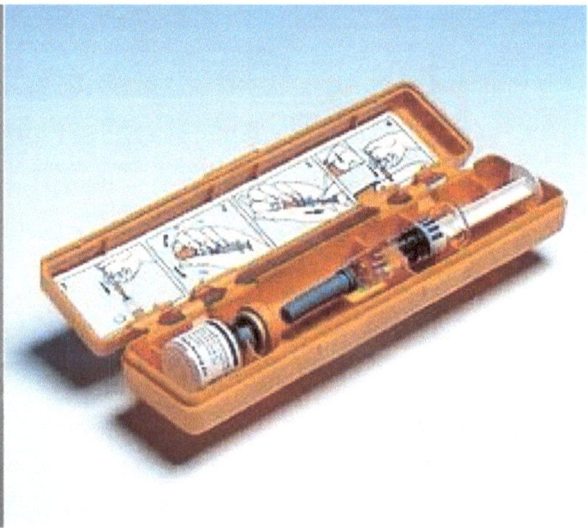

Glucagon Emergency Kit

Glucogen HypoKit

Dizziness or Vertigo

Dizziness/vertigo can be frightening to patients and frustrating to physicians because of the difficulty in accurately diagnosing the etiology of the disorder. In the workplace it is important to rule out exposures at work as the source of dizziness/vertigo, as this will be helpful to the managing physician in his differential diagnosis. History should, therefore, attempt to describe whether the incidents are related to activities in the workplace.

Treatment:

For complaints of dizziness or vertigo:

1. Obtain a brief work history to include onset, duration, relieving and aggravating factors, social history to include smoking and alcohol use, prior episodes of dizziness or vertigo, etc.

2. Take blood pressure.

3. Check pupillary response.

4. If symptoms do not subside in a period of 15-20 minutes, the patient should be referred for evaluation by a physician and not allowed to return to work without a physician's permission.

5. Associated symptoms requiring a physician evaluation: difficulty with vision, difficulty with speech, weakness and numbness.

Domestic Abuse / Violence (Real or Suspected)

Domestic Violence

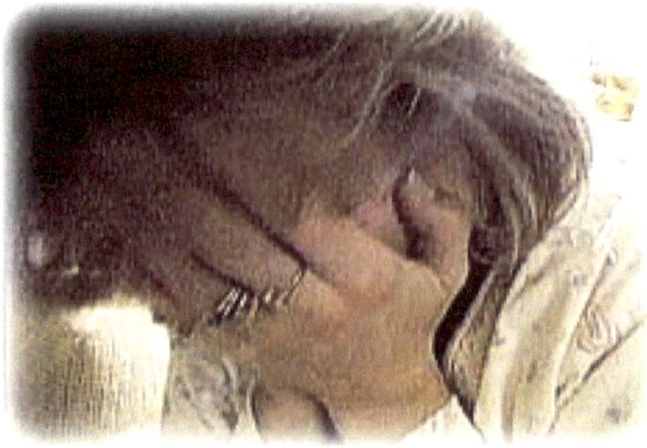

Domestic violence is a pattern of assaultive and coercive behaviors, including physical, sexual, and psychological attacks, as well as economic coercion, that adults or adolescents use against their intimate partner.

Domestic violence is:

- A pattern of behaviors including a variety of tactics – some physically injurious and some not, some criminal and some not – carried out in multiple, sometimes daily episodes.
- A combination of physical force and terror used by the perpetrator that causes physical and psychological harm to the victim and children.
- A pattern of purposeful behavior directed at achieving compliance from or control over the victim.
- Behaviors perpetrated by adults or adolescents against their intimate partner in current or former dating, married, or cohabiting relationships of heterosexuals, gays and lesbians

If you become aware of any case (or suspected case) of domestic abuse:

1. Encourage employee to call the local agency on Sexual Assault and Domestic Violence:

   Agency: ______________________________

   Phone: ________________________________

2. Follow-up with employee on next onsite visit or per phone.

Ear Difficulty

Introduction:

A common source of ear problems in the workplace relates to work in a noisy environment. Improperly worn hearing protection devices, other forms of trauma, along with infection (which may be work-related) are sources of problems with the ear.

Treatment:

1. Obtain history and vital signs.

2. With use of the otoscope, check the ear canal for obvious problems related to disease or to trauma, perhaps from improperly used hearing protection devices.

3. For signs or symptoms of infection, such as fever, rhinorrhea, lymphadenopathy, possible bulging eardrum and/or perforated eardrum, refer to a physician for evaluation and treatment. Otherwise, may give acetaminophen (Tylenol) 500 mg 1-2 tablets every 6 hours PRN. If unsure, refer to a company physician for evaluation and treatment.

4. For signs of ear wax (ceruminosis), may use OTC ear wax treatment such as Debrox. Refer to physician for cerumen impaction not improved with OTC treatment.

Environmental Allergies

Environmental allergies, also known as hay fever, can create significant problems for workers who spend time in the outdoors. Symptoms can include watery eyes, runny nose, post-nasal drainage, a feeling of swollen eyes or nose or mild cough. It is important to differentiate common allergies from anaphylactic shock (please see that section regarding that condition).

Hay fever is an allergic reaction. It is your immune system's response to foreign material in the air you breathe. Hay fever usually refers to allergies to outdoor, airborne materials such as pollens and molds.

About 15-20% of the population of the United States has some degree of hay fever. It is found equally in both men and women. Usually hay fever is seasonal, but it can last all year long if the allergen stays throughout the year. Spring and fall are the main hay fever seasons.

Most allergy sufferers are familiar with their symptoms and many will self-medicate. As previously prescription-only medications have become over the counter preparations, this has helped dramatically. However, caution should be taken if the symptoms continue or worsen despite utilization of these medications.

Treatment:

Avoid known or suspected allergens.

Gargle with warm salt water, 1-2 tablespoons of table salt in 8 ounces of warm water, to soothe a mildly sore throat.

Take nonprescription antihistamines to relieve symptoms of sneezing, runny nose, and itchy throat and eyes. Caution - these medications may make you too drowsy to drive a car or operate machinery safely.

For stuffy nose, a combination of an antihistamine and a decongestant.

Reasonable OTC medications that may be administered in an onsite environment include:

Decongestants:

Pseudoephedrine 30 to 60 mg every 4 to 6 hours

Oxymetazoline nasal spray every 12 hours (should not exceed 2-3 days of use)

Anti-histamines:

Diphenhydramine 25 mg every 4 to 6 hours as needed;
do not exceed 150 mg/day

Loratadine 10 mg every day as needed

Fexofenadine 60 mg every 12 hours as needed

Cetirizine 10 mg every day as needed

If symptoms persist despite treatment, referral to a physician is warranted.

The occupational health nurse should be aware and review with the worker any potential side effects from these medications and be aware and communicate any drug-drug interactions that may be of concern. Always consult the package insert for this information.

Eye Conditions

Introduction:

Any complaint of irritation, injury, or foreign body suspected in the eye should be seen as soon as possible to determine cause and treatment.

Treatment:

Chemical Irritation in the Eye:

1. Most chemicals are irritating to the eye.

2. The initial step to treatment of any chemical in the eye is immediate irrigation with copious amounts of water. This irrigation should start ***before*** the patient arrives at the nursing station.

3. The eye should be thoroughly irrigated by the nurse until transported to physician or emergency room.

4. These patients should then be referred to the company physician or ophthalmologist.

Flash Burns of the Eye:

1. Eyes that are exposed to severe ultraviolet radiation, such as occurs with welding, may develop a keratoconjunctivitis (welder's flash).

2. Onset is usually 4-6 hours after exposure, commencing with a sandy, gritty sensation in the eye, intense sensitivity to light, tearing and pain.

3. Flash burns are usually bilateral and self-limited, clearing in 48 hours.

4. Flash burns may be aided by cold compresses and patching in some cases.

5. All cases should be referred to the company physician and/or ophthalmologist.

Foreign Bodies to the Eye:

Introduction:

The most common eye injury in industry is a foreign body. Most metallic foreign bodies are located in the conjunctival sac.

Treatment:

1. Examine the eye under bright light with magnification.

2. If the foreign body is seen, attempts should be made to irrigate it out with copious amounts of water.

3. If this is not successful, the foreign body may be touched with a sterile applicator that has been moistened with sterile water or eye irrigating solution. A light touch should be used to avoid producing a corneal abrasion. Care should be taken not to rub or further embed the foreign body.

4. If the above measures are unsuccessful, the eye should be patched, and the patient referred to the company physician or ophthalmologist.

Conjunctivitis

Conjunctivitis is an inflammation of the conjunctiva characterized by cellular infiltration and exudation. Symptoms may include:

1. Diffuse gritty, foreign body sensation in the eye.

2. Exudation.

3. Burning sensation.

4. Redness, "irritated" look.

5. Photophobia.

<u>Treatment</u>:

1. A clinical course of conjunctivitis may last 2-3 weeks and is relatively easy to transmit by contact with discharges from the eye or upper respiratory tract of infected person.

2. Refer to physician for evaluation.

Fainting / Syncope

Introduction:

An individual who faints while in the workplace should be evaluated by a physician prior to returning to work. An attempt should be made while taking the history to determine if the episode was related to the workplace.

Treatment:

1. Loosen the clothing and provide fresh air.

2. Attempt to determine the history of the episode including employee's activities prior to fainting. Also inquire about any previous episodes of loss of consciousness.

3. Have the employee remain flat.

4. Monitor vital signs. May ***cautiously*** use an ammonia inhalant PRN. Do not use ammonia inhalant close than 4" to 6" from the patient's face.

5. This employee should be referred to a physician or emergency room accompanied by another responsible person.

Fever

Introduction:

Fever is usually a sign of infectious disease. However, it should be remembered that elevated body temperature is also a sign of hyperthermia, which may occur commonly in some workplaces. Some chemical exposures may cause an elevated core temperature as well. As such, a high index of suspicion should be maintained, and an accurate history is important to define the exact etiology.

Treatment:

1. Temperature elevation should be verified by a temperature recording by the Occupational Health nurse.

2. If temperature is 99.6 or above, advise employee concerning options. For mild fever, acetaminophen or ibuprofen can be taken. For higher fevers, or if mild fevers with other constitutional symptoms, advise the patient to go home and advise to see own doctor if no improvement in 1-2 days. Follow-up with employee per phone in 1-2 days.

3. If hyperthermia or chemical exposure is determined to be the etiology of an elevated body temperature, treat as noted in the appropriate sections of these guidelines.

4. The employee should be afebrile for 24 hours prior to returning to work. Depending on the client's company, a return-to-work form from the patient's physician may be necessary.

Fractures and Dislocations

Introduction:

Fractures and dislocations must be treated appropriately in the field setting.

Treatment:

1. Check CAB's, control bleeding, prevent contamination while awaiting transportation.

2. Check circulation and neurovascular status distal to injury and check for the classic signs of arterial insufficiency: decreased or absent pulse, paleness, paresthesia, pain and paralysis.

3. Immobilize the fractured or dislocated part with splints, as appropriate. Provide support above ***and*** below the affected joint.

4. Arrange for an immediate transfer to an emergency facility. (Some company physicians have x-ray and fracture care capabilities in their office. A phone call will identify those who do.)

5. Keep patient NPO.

6. Tips on applying a splint: splint most injuries "as they lie" except when the neurovascular status is compromised. Secure the splint to the injured extremity with straps or gauze. Do not use elastic bandage.

Frostbite / Hypothermia

Introduction:

The severity of cold injuries depends on the ambient temperature, duration of exposure, and environmental conditions. Lower temperature, immobilization, prolonged exposure, moisture, the presence of peripheral vascular disease, and open wounds all increase the severity of the injury. Three types of cold injuries are seen:

- Frostbite
- Non-freezing injury, due to prolonged exposure over several days
- Hypothermia

Signs of frostbite include redness or discoloration of the affected part. It may be cold, hard, and white then cold and blotchy red, swollen and painful as tissue is warmed.

Treatment:

Management of Frostbite and Non-Freezing Cold Injuries

1. ***Treatment should be immediate*** to decrease duration of tissue freezing.

2. Damp, cold clothing should be replaced by warm blankets.

3. Warm the frostbitten area in ***lukewarm*** or ***tepid*** water (100-105 degrees). Do not use hot water.

4. The patient should be given hot fluids by mouth, if able to drink.

5. Elevate the affected extremity if possible.

6. ***Do not rub*** the skin.

7. Refer to physician for evaluation.

8. Inquire as to tetanus immunization status. If required, follow the tetanus immunization protocol.

Management of Hypothermia

Hypothermia may be classified as mild (body temperature of 32-35º centigrade), moderate (30-31º centigrade), or severe (below 30º centigrade).

Signs of hypothermia would include a depressed level of consciousness, the most common feature of hypothermia. The patient is cold to touch and appears gray and cyanotic.

1. Follow the CAB's. This should include initiation of CPR if necessary.
2. Treat ***mild hypothermia by passive external re-warming*** in a warm room using warm blankets and clothing.
3. Activate Emergency Medical Services (**911**) system.
4. In instances where a cold, injured patient may appear to be clinically dead, it is important to remember that **<u>NO PATIENT IS DEAD, UNTIL THEY ARE WARM AND DEAD</u>.**

Gastrointestinal Distress

Introduction:

There are many sources of gastrointestinal distress in the workplace. Some chemical exposures, as well as irritable bowel syndrome induced by stress, as well as gastroenteritis, may be sources of abdominal pain. It is, therefore, important to obtain an accurate history.

Treatment:

1. Obtain history of complaint.

2. Any history of severe pain in the abdomen, vomiting, uncontrolled diarrhea, or fever should be seen by a physician as soon as possible.

3. Vital signs including temperature as indicated.

4. If complaint appears to be a minor GI upset, may use the following:

   - For heartburn, may give Maalox two Tablespoons by mouth QID; Antacids such as Mylanta, Tums, or Rolaids can also be helpful. Antacids work by neutralizing acid. They should be taken 1 hour after meals or when heartburn symptoms occur.

     Low doses of drugs that block the production of stomach acid are available over-the-counter. Some examples include cimetidine (Tagamet), ranitidine (Zantac), and famotidine (Pepcid) and omeprazole (Prilosec OTC).

   - For diarrhea, may give bismuth subsalicylate (Pepto-Bismol®) 1-2 Tablespoons after each diarrheal stool or loperamide HCl (Imodium®) as directed. If symptoms persist longer than 7-10 days, refer patient to physician.

5. Diarrhea caused by viral infections typically ends on its own without antibiotics. Over-the-counter (OTC) medications may slow diarrhea, but they won't speed your recovery. Certain infections may be made worse by OTC medications because they prevent your body from getting rid of what's causing the diarrhea.

Headache

There are many types of headaches. The most common are muscle tension type headaches and those that associated with infections. It can be difficult to differentiate the cause of headaches, especially those that are recurrent or chronic, and often are "mixed", meaning that they arise from multiple sources.

Treatment:

1. Check blood pressure.

2. Obtain history:

    - If accompanied by dizziness, nausea, vomiting, stiff neck, history of recurrence, general malaise, or other symptoms, employee should be referred.

    - Headache may be caused by exposure to toxic substances on the job or may be indicative of other illnesses.

3. If headache appears uncomplicated: Aspirin 325mg every 4 hours as needed, acetaminophen 500 mg two tablets every 4-6 hours as needed, ibuprofen 200 mg two tablets every 8 hours as needed, or naproxen sodium 220 mg one or two tablets every 12 hours as needed.

4. Advise employee to return to the health service if unrelieved.

Head Injury

Introduction:

All moderate or severe head injuries, especially where unconsciousness occurs, should be referred to a physician for evaluation.

Treatment:

1. Monitor CAB's.
2. Activate Emergency Medical Services (**911**) system.
3. Monitor vital signs including pupil reaction.
4. Control bleeding, if applicable.
5. Suspect neck injury and avoid further damage by immobilizing.
6. Keep patient quiet, with head slightly elevated.
7. Keep patient NPO.
8. Notify emergency room that will receive patient.

Heat Reactions

Heat Cramps

<u>Introduction</u>:

Heat cramps usually occur when a person is doing hard work in hot weather and drinking great volumes of water. This causes the dilution of electrolytes in addition to electrolyte loss from excessive perspiration.

<u>Treatment</u>:

- Rest
- Cool environment
- Fluid replacement in the form of electrolytes replacement (i.e., Gatorade / Powerade / All-Sport) is preferable. If not available, water may be used.
- Salt tablets should be discouraged

Heat Exhaustion

<u>Introduction</u>:

Heat exhaustion occurs when there is a prolonged period of fluid loss (i.e., from perspiration, diarrhea, or use of diuretics) and exposure to warm ambient temperatures without adequate fluid and electrolyte replacement.

Symptoms:

- Normal, subnormal or mildly elevated temperature
- Dizziness
- Nausea/vomiting
- Weakness
- Pallor
- Headache
- Pulse can be slow or rapid

<u>Treatment</u>:

- Rest
- Cool environment and loosen clothing
- If conscious, give sips of water (or Gatorade)
- If vomits, do not give more fluids
- Monitor vital signs
- Transport for further care

Heat Stroke

Introduction:

Heat stroke is an emergency which may be precipitated by hot environment, exercise, or certain medications. Death will occur if body temperature is not lowered, because the body will have lost its ability to dissipate heat.

Symptoms:

- Temperature may be up to 105 degrees F.
- Hot, dry skin
- Dizziness
- Flushed face
- Decreasing level of consciousness
- Rapid pulse
- Confusion, coma or convulsions

Treatment:

- Remove patient to cool environment.
- Activate Emergency Medical Services (**911**) system.
- Monitor CAB's.
- Attempt to reduce body temperature by cold compresses to head, groin and wrists. Cooling blankets may be utilized.
- Anticipate possible cardiac arrest due to electrolyte imbalance.

Hernia

Introduction:

Characterized by swelling in the groin (inguinal), around the belly button (umbilical) or in other parts of the abdomen (abdominal wall). Possible severe pain may occur after muscular effort.

Treatment:

1. Have patient lie on back with knees bent.

2. Obtain history regarding onset and related circumstances, which may determine if work-related.

3. Arrange for physician evaluation.

4. Advise patient ***no lifting*** until seen by physician.

Impaired Worker

- If an employee is suspected to be under the influence of alcohol and/or drugs, consult with company contact person for individual company policy.
- Provide assistance to company and employee as needed. For additional information, contact local addiction/recovery agency.

*If employer is an EAP client, contact EAP for further information and scheduling.

**If employer is not an EAP client, but crisis intervention is indicated, refer to appropriate emergency department/service.

Employee Assistance Program: ______________________________

EAP Phone: ______________________________

Information Technology / Smartphone / Small Tablet PC

<u>Introduction:</u>

A quiet revolution has been going on in the medical profession and the field of personal health in the last several years, spearheaded by smartphones and tablets that will change forever the way we obtain and process medical information. Occupational health nurses, oftentimes in providing services to industry in remote locations, have found these devices helpful in many ways.

Occupational Health Nursing Applications:

1. Digital photography for documentation of burns, rashes, lacerations, scars etc.
2. Video clips used for documentation of ROM, gait etc.
3. Database creation and access
4. Educational access (there are a wide variety of health education applications available for download)
5. Communication with health care providers.

Confidentiality and Information Protection:

The occupational health nurse is encouraged to use smartphone and iPad technology for the purposes stated above when appropriate. Transmission of digital photographs can be quite useful to physicians and other health care providers. These communications can also be used within the larger scope of telemedicine.

It should be understood that photographs and other medical data that are stored within these devices are protected pieces of medical information. Once transmitted to the end-user, the digital data, whether it is a photograph, video clip or written data should be erased from the device's memory.

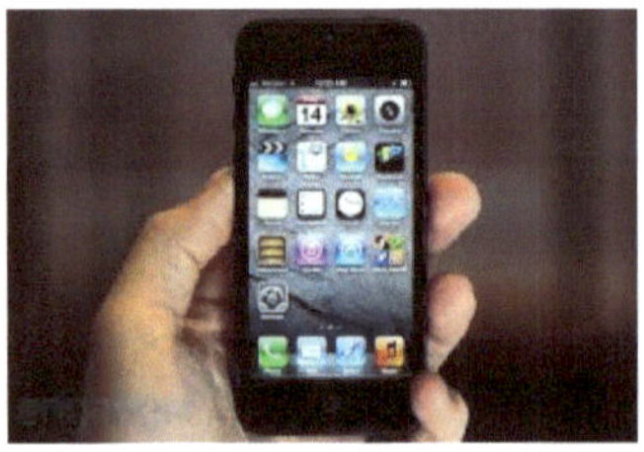

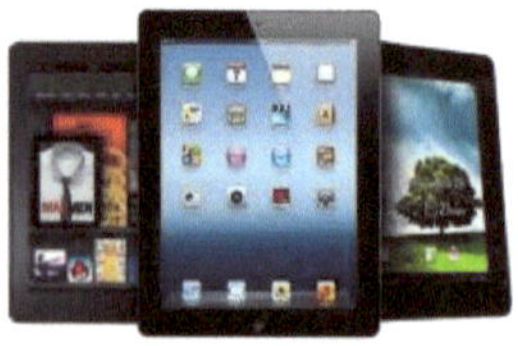

Injection Injuries

Introduction:

Injection injuries are one of the subtlest, yet most serious injuries that can occur in an industrial setting. Any history of an employee having suffered a high-pressured injection injury requires that the employee be referred as quickly as possible for more definitive medical care. Injection of paints and oils, for example, produces a serious problem that requires immediate attention.

Treatment:

1. Any injection injury should be seen ***as soon as possible*** by the company physician for appropriate treatment.
2. Keep limb lower than heart level.
3. Check for pulses in arm/wrist.
4. Apply cool/ice packs to injury site and refer to physician.

Lacerations

Introduction:

All lacerations should be cleansed thoroughly with antibacterial soap and water (preferred) or Betadine scrub. Many can be closed by the nurse with a butterfly dressing, also known as steri-strips. Mastisol® (or similar) liquid adhesive can provide better adherence of these types of dressings. Control bleeding with direct pressure with sterile gauze.

Treatment:

The patient should be referred to a physician if:

- The laceration is more than minor in degree and cannot be easily closed, such as a deep or gaping laceration.
- Facial laceration.
- If located over a joint.
- The wound appears infected; i.e., warmth, redness, purulent drainage, excessive soreness.
- Possible nerve/tendon involvement. In this case, keep the patient NPO.
- Inquire as to tetanus status (see Tetanus Immunization Directive).
- Instruct patient in wound care.

Nosebleed (Epistaxis)

Introduction:

Most instances of nosebleed occur from the anterior portion of the nose along the septum. Causes include trauma, foreign bodies, hypertension, hematologic disturbances, and very rarely, nasal tumors.

Treatment:

1. Apply cold packs to the bridge of the nose.

2. Pinch both nostrils closed with firm, gentle pressure for 5 minutes. Have the patient tilt head forward.

3. If bleeding is stopped by the above, have the patient sit up and advise him/her not to blow through the nose for 1-2 hours after.

4. If bleeding is severe or is not controlled in 10 minutes, arrange for the patient to be seen by physician.

5. Recurrent nosebleeds, or nosebleeds that fail to resolve with conservative treatment may indicate other problems, such as hypertension or clotting abnormalities. Please refer such patient to physician for further evaluation.

Oxygen Therapy

Not every occupational health nursing department will be equipped with supplemental oxygen. A determination of the suitability for the provision and use of oxygen for therapeutic purposes is driven by a wide variety of factors.

Guidelines for oxygen therapy are per the ER/Trauma protocol. Many times, the flow rate will be determined by the caregiver at the scene. For most severe chest pain, traumatic injury or shock, a non-rebreather mask will provide the most relief for an injured person (if they can tolerate the mask).

General outlines for oxygen administration are:

- 2 L/cannula – person with COPD or emphysema
- 6 L/cannula – mild to moderate discomfort
- 12-15 L/non-rebreather – pulmonary irritant
- 12-15 L/non-rebreather – traumatic injury
- 12-15 L/non-rebreather – severe chest pain

The Occupational Heath nurses' role is to help stabilize a person until EMS personnel arrive to assist.

Pharyngitis (Sore Throat)

Background:

Pharyngitis is defined as an infection or irritation of the pharynx and/or tonsils. The etiology is usually infectious, with 40-60% of cases being of viral origin and 5-40% of cases being of bacterial origin. Other causes include allergy, trauma, toxins, and neoplasia.

The main concerns with pharyngitis are to rule out more serious conditions, such as epiglottitis or peritonsillar abscess, and to diagnose group A beta-hemolytic streptococcal (GABHS) infections. GABHS infections can have serious sequelae and represent approximately 15% of all physician pharyngitis visits.

Evaluation:

- Airway patency must be addressed first.
- Temperature
    - Fever is usually absent or low-grade in viral pharyngitis, but this is not specific enough to differentiate viral and bacterial etiologies.
    - Fever can be as high as 106°F with coxsackievirus A, coxsackievirus B, herpes simplex, GABHS infection, HIV-1, infectious mononucleosis, and cytomegalovirus (CMV).
- Hydration status: Oral intake usually is compromised because of odynophagia; therefore, various degrees of dehydration result.
- HEENT
    - Conjunctivitis may be seen in association with adenovirus.
    - Scleral icterus may be seen with infectious mononucleosis.
    - Rhinorrhea usually is associated with a viral cause.

- Tonsillopharyngeal/palatal petechiae are seen in GABHS infections and infectious mononucleosis.

- A tonsillopharyngeal exudate may be seen in streptococcal infectious mononucleosis and occasionally in *M pneumoniae, C pneumoniae, A haemolyticus*, adenovirus, and herpesvirus infections. Therefore, exudate does not differentiate viral and bacterial causes.

a) Oropharyngeal vesicular lesions are seen in coxsackievirus and herpesvirus. Concomitant vesicles on the hands and feet are associated with coxsackievirus (hand-foot-and-mouth disease).

- Lymphadenopathy: Tender anterior cervical nodes are consistent with streptococcal infection, while generalized adenopathy is consistent with infectious mononucleosis or the acute lymphoglandular syndrome of HIV infection.

Treatment:

- Lozenges (cough medicine) are often used for short-term pain relief.
- Gargling with warm salty water is a popular household remedy, although there is only anecdotal evidence this gives other than temporary relief and likewise for the use of aspirin gargles.
- Warm tea can help temporarily alleviate the pain of a sore throat.
- Analgesics such as NSAIDs can help reduce the pain associated with a sore throat.
- Refer to physician for severe symptoms or symptoms that persist beyond 48 hours.

Poisoning

Introduction:

Poisonings that occur in the workplace may be insidious as well as obvious to the casual observer. Workplace toxicity may develop acutely from overexposure in high doses or may occur on a more chronic basis secondary to recurring, low-dose exposure, as occurred with the radium watch dial painters in 1950's England. Knowing the source of poison is helpful to Poison Control Center and EMS people. ***Encourage companies to have SDS sheets available and up to date on products in the company.***

Treatment:

Inhaled

1. Remove to fresh air.

2. Give oxygen (5-6 L) and CPR if necessary.

3. Active Emergency Medical Services (911) system.

4. Vital signs.

5. Exercise extreme caution in removing victim from an area with a toxic atmosphere. **IT IS IMPORTANT TO AVOID BECOMING A VICTIM YOURSELF.**

6. Notify trauma center receiving patient of situation.

Surface

1. Remove from source.

2. Remove clothing contaminated with poison.

3. Flush with water for several minutes.

Ingested

1. Quickly gather information on substance ingested; i.e., label, name, SDS sheet.

2. Call Poison Control regarding antidote and emergency care (or immediate transfer to hospital).

   Poison Control Center Phone: ______________________________

3. Do not induce vomiting, if the patient is unconscious, seizing, or has ingested acid, alkali or petroleum products. Have the following available: Syrup of Ipecac and activated charcoal. **DO NOT USE THESE WITHOUT THE ADVICE OF A POISON CONTROL CENTER.**

4. After following the advice of the physician in the Poison Control Center, transport to a hospital.

Pregnancy

Introduction:

Questioning of women routinely concerning the possibility of pregnancy should eliminate the error of giving medications to women in early pregnancy or who may be pregnant.

Treatment:

When a woman is known to be pregnant or suspects pregnancy, no medication should be given to that individual without prior approval from a physician.

It is also important to ask a pregnant woman concerning her workplace, as this may reveal a potential reproductive hazard by exposure or by other sources.

Should a work site reproductive hazard be identified, consultation should be obtained with the Medical Director.

Pulmonary Irritants

Introduction:

There are many potential respiratory irritants that can be encountered in the industrial setting. The occupational health nurse should investigate common potential agents within the facility they are working with and gain some familiarity with common medical issues that can arise. Emergency treatment for acute exposure to many irritants may be necessary.

Diagnostic concerns:

1. Get exposure history – intensity, duration and chemical name from safety data sheets.

2. Get patient's medical history for symptoms of respiratory tract and mucosal irritation:

    Lacrimation; rhinitis; sore, dry or burning throat; cough; chest tightness; chest burning; shortness of breath; and/or difficulty breathing.

3. Get patient's history for nonspecific symptoms such as headache, muscle cramps, nausea, vomiting, dizziness, and/or syncope.

4. Physical assessment should include vital sign measurements. If full trained, equipped and under medical supervision, chest auscultation and pulmonary function test can be done.

Treatment:

1. Remove immediately from exposure area.

2. Monitor vital signs and be prepared to administer CPR, if needed.

3. Administer oxygen at 12-15L/minute with non-rebreather mask (if can tolerate mask).

4. Rest elevate legs and cover with blanket if evidence of shock.

5. Consult a physician as soon as practical or send directly to nearest emergency room if:

    a. Patient's condition deteriorates rapidly, and/or
    b. Physician cannot be contacted.

6. Record details of exposure and patient's findings and course while under your care. Forward this information to treating physician.

7. Remind physician of possibility of delayed onset of pulmonary edema if moderate to high-level exposure.

Respiratory Inflammation/Infection

Introduction:

The respiratory system's defenses against particle inhalation can be grouped into three lines of defense successively encountered by particles that enter the airways.

The first line of defense is the progressive mechanical filtering through the upper airways and the lower airways. The second line of defense is provided by the fluids that line the airways and gas exchanging structures and by the clearance mechanisms that physically remove particles from their surfaces. The last line of defense is composed of the specific immunological defenses of the lung brought into play against biochemically active particles that deposit in the lung. These lines of defense are interdependent and coordinated as well.

Should a patient present with symptoms or respiratory irritation, infection or difficulty in breathing, it is important to obtain a thorough history. Questions should include a history of the incident, including location. Other historical areas of importance include whether the individual was wearing a respirator and to what potential intoxicants the employee may have been exposed to that could produce any respiratory symptoms. It is important to remember that the onset of respiratory symptoms may be delayed for 24-48 hours after a toxic respiratory exposure. Pay attention to whether carbon monoxide, hydrogen sulfide or hydrogen cyanide exposures could have occurred.

Treatment:

1. Check vital signs. Commence oxygen therapy, if the patient has any evidence of respiratory impairment. Remember that oxygen may depress respiratory drive in some patients with COPD. An accurate history is critical.

2. Examine the eyes, nose and pharynx for any evidence of chemical or thermal burns. Should this evidence be present, refer immediately to the emergency room.

3. Carefully auscultate the lungs for the presence of rhonchi or rales. Listen over the larynx or tracheal for an inspiratory stridor, which is best heard when the subject makes a rapid respiratory effort.

4. For evidence of significant respiratory distress, refer to the emergency room for further treatment.

5. If respiratory irritation appears to be mild, and/or the patient has symptoms of an upper respiratory tract infection, the following suggestions may be tried:

   - For cold symptoms, a decongestant may be recommended, such as pseudoephedrine 30 mg every 4 hours PRN or phenylephrine 10 mg every 4 hours PRN if there are no contraindications, such as blood pressure, diabetes or heart disease. If symptoms persist longer than 7-10 days, patient should be advised to consult with their personal physician.

   - Cough may be treated with Robitussin DM 10 cc every 4 hours PRN if indicated.

   - For sore throat, lozenges or saline gargles may be used.

   - The intent of this therapy is **NOT** to provide definitive treatment. Rather it is to get the employee through the shift so they may see their own private physician.

   - Always refer a patient to their personal physician.

Sexual Assault

If an employee confides or reports to you a case of sexual assault, including rape:

1. ***Strongly*** encourage the person to contact the appropriate local agency for sexual assault for assistance or refer directly to law enforcement or medical center. The local agency will take necessary steps to assist employee to contact law enforcement and arrange medical care.

   Local sexual assault assistance agency: ____________________________

   Phone: ______________________________________

   Law Enforcement Phone: _____________________

2. Follow-up with employee on next onsite visit or per phone.

3. Instruct person to not shower or bathe until examination is carried out.

Shock Protocol

Introduction:

Shock is a clinical state resulting from inadequate tissue perfusion. Alterations in the sensorium are characteristic of the shock state. Anxiety, restlessness, fear, apathy, stupor or coma may be present. These abnormalities reflect diminished cerebral perfusion.

Treatment:

1. Active Emergency Medical Services (911) system.
2. Monitor patient's CAB's.
3. Keep the patient warm, dry and on his/her back with feet slightly elevated. Do not elevate feet in case of a) head injury, b) back injury, c) breathing difficulty increased, or d) complaints of pain when attempted.
4. Monitor vital signs.
5. Oxygen at high flow rate.
6. Stay with person until emergency help arrives.

Splinters

Treatment:

1. Cleanse with Betadine scrub (soap and water are also okay).

2. Attempt to remove with tweezers or forceps or scrape with straight edge.

3. If other than superficially lodged, or not able to remove entire splinter, refer to physician for removal.

4. After removal, apply Betadine ointment or antibiotic ointment and clean dressing.

5. Check tetanus status.

Sprains, Strains and other Musculoskeletal System Disorders

Introduction:

The diagnosis, treatment and rehabilitation of musculoskeletal disorders constitute a large portion of clinical occupational medical practice. The health professional that provides occupational medical services is likely to encounter strains, especially to the neck, back and shoulder. Repetitive motion injuries, also called cumulative trauma disorders include such conditions as tendinitis, myositis, fasciitis, and others.

As for any medical problem, it is important to obtain the history. The history should include such pertinent items as patient's normal job, length and duration of symptoms, aggravating or relieving factors, etc.

- **Strain** – A strain is an overstretching of a muscle or group of muscles in such a way that the microscopic individual bundles making up the muscle are torn or the tendon, by which the muscle is fostered to the bone which it moves, is stretched or ruptured.

- **Sprain** – Sprains are injuries to the ligaments about a joint, or to the joint covering (capsule) itself, which produce undue stretching or actual tearing of these tissues.

Treatment:

Extremity (Acute Sprains/Strains):

1. Rest and elevate the injured part, applying cold packs for 15-20 minutes every 2-3 hours.

2. Apply ACE or similar bandage to the injured part.

3. Should the individual be unable to bear weight on an injured knee, ankle or foot, gross swelling or discoloration, refer to the company physician for appropriate evaluation for possible fracture.

4. If no evidence of a fracture is present (i.e., gross swelling, deformity, tenderness, discoloration, decreased ROM, inability to bear weight), recheck with the patient in 2-3 days or advise patient to notify the Occupational Health nurse or office if symptoms worsen or become severe.

5. If any doubt, send for evaluation with physician.

6. Instruct patient on home care.

Low Back Pain:

<u>Introduction</u>:

Low back pain the number one disorder that will be encountered by the occupational health nurse and is the most common diagnosis seen within an occupational medicine clinic. It has been stated that low back pain is so common, that it might be more correct to discuss that it is a normal part of the human condition as opposed to a health calamity. The good news is that 90% of all cases of acute low back pain will resolve relatively quickly regardless of cause, even if only minimal medical treatment is given.

<u>Evaluation:</u>

- Obtain an adequate history. An accurate history is necessary to determine the origin of the employee's discomfort, which may or may not be occupational in nature. This should be directed to the onset of pain, its character, duration, radiation and measures that relieve the discomfort. Questions regarding symptoms such as pain radiation especially down the posterior aspect of the leg, numbness and paresthesia of the feet or weakness can help determine whether nerve root irritation secondary to a possible herniated disk is present. It is also helpful to inquire about the nature of the work that the person performs, including the availability of mechanical lifting devices and the weight of the material that is expected to be lifted. Questions should be directed to rule out other causes of back pain, including spondylolisthesis, cancer and obesity.

- Complete an ergonomic work site assessment to determine and review causational factors. This is to include a review of the types of motions and movements, force and lifting factors, and the level of repetitive work. Video recording of the work type might be beneficial in some circumstances.

- Physical examination should include an observation of the patient walking. ROM should be recorded. Paraspinal muscle spasms should be noted. Both seated and supine straight leg raising should be performed.

Treatment:

1. For mild-to-moderate back pain:

    - Give ibuprofen up to 800 mg every 8 hours for pain and swelling, unless contraindicated, or Aleve® (naproxen sodium) 220-440 mg 2 times/day, or Orudis KT® (ketoprofen) 12.5 mg – 25 mg once daily. This may be given for 5-7 days. If pain is still unrelieved, refer to a physician.

    - Use an ice pack for 15-20 minutes every 2-3 hours daily for 3 days. Some patients also will benefit from heat applications of the same duration. If symptoms persist, refer to physician.

    - Appropriate modified / transitional duty may be instituted by the onsite nurse. In general, mild-to-moderate back pain should not be a reason for restricted duty. Every attempt should be made to return the employee to his/her regular duties whenever possible. It is unlikely that an employee will need to be restricted beyond a 20 lb. material handling limit for mild-to-moderate back pain. Evidence based research clearly shows that early return to normal activities provides the best long-term outcome for low back pain.

    - Follow-up with patient in 1-2 days.

2. Refer to company physician for:

- Severe back pain.
- Any radicular signs; i.e., pain shooting into leg.
- Any neurological signs; i.e., difficulty urinating, defecating, numbness, weakness of lower extremities.

3. Reassurance given to the patient is paramount. Remember that 90% of all back pain will be relieved within four weeks regardless of cause and treatment.

Cumulative Trauma Disorders

Introduction:

A good management program that seeks to identify early and treat these important disorders quickly is important. The following systematic approach to evaluating, treating and following workers who report to the health facility is recommended:

- CTD screening assessment by occupational health nurse. This will include obtaining a history and an ergonomic work site assessment to determine review of causational factors. This is to include review of type of motions and movements, force and lifting factors, and level of repetitive work. A brief screening examination for the evaluation of CTD consists of inspection, palpation, ROM testing and various provocative maneuvers.

- New and transferred employees should be given the opportunity during a six-week break-in period to condition their muscle tendon groups prior to working at full capacity. These employees should have a follow-up assessment after the break-in period to determine if conditioning of the muscle tendon groups has been successful. If problems are identified, further action is required, such as 1) extend break-in period for two weeks, or 2) CTD assessment with follow-up.

Treatment:

1. See written protocols for CTD guidelines.

2. Splints that may be used are night time finger extension splints, Proflex (or similar) wrist splints, cock-up splints, tennis elbow straps or Comfort Cool (or similar) thumb spica splints. Other splints may be approved on an individual basis upon consultation with the medical director.

3. Give Ibuprofen up to 800 mg q 8 hours or Aleve® 220-440 mg q 8-12 hours, Orudis KT® (ketoprofen) 12.5 – 25 mg q day. Aspirin 1 or 2 tabs every 8 hours as a substitute for these NSAIDs. If there is a contraindication to NSAID's, acetaminophen Tylenol ES® two tablets every 4-6 hours may be given as an alternative.

4. If an employee misses a scheduled re-evaluation, the nurse should contact the employee to assess the condition within approximately five days of the last presentation.

5. Refer to company physician or healthcare provider according to written protocols for CTD.

6. The referring physicians or healthcare providers should be furnished with a written description of the ergonomic characteristics of the job of the worker who is being referred.

7. When an employee returns to work after time off to rest an inflamed tendon, ligament or nerve, there must be reconditioning of the healing muscle tendon groups. Consideration should be given to permanently reassigning the worker to an available job with the lower risk of developing CTD's.

8. Be aware of OSHA Recordkeeping Guidelines for Occupational Illnesses (CTD's).

CTD Symptom Management

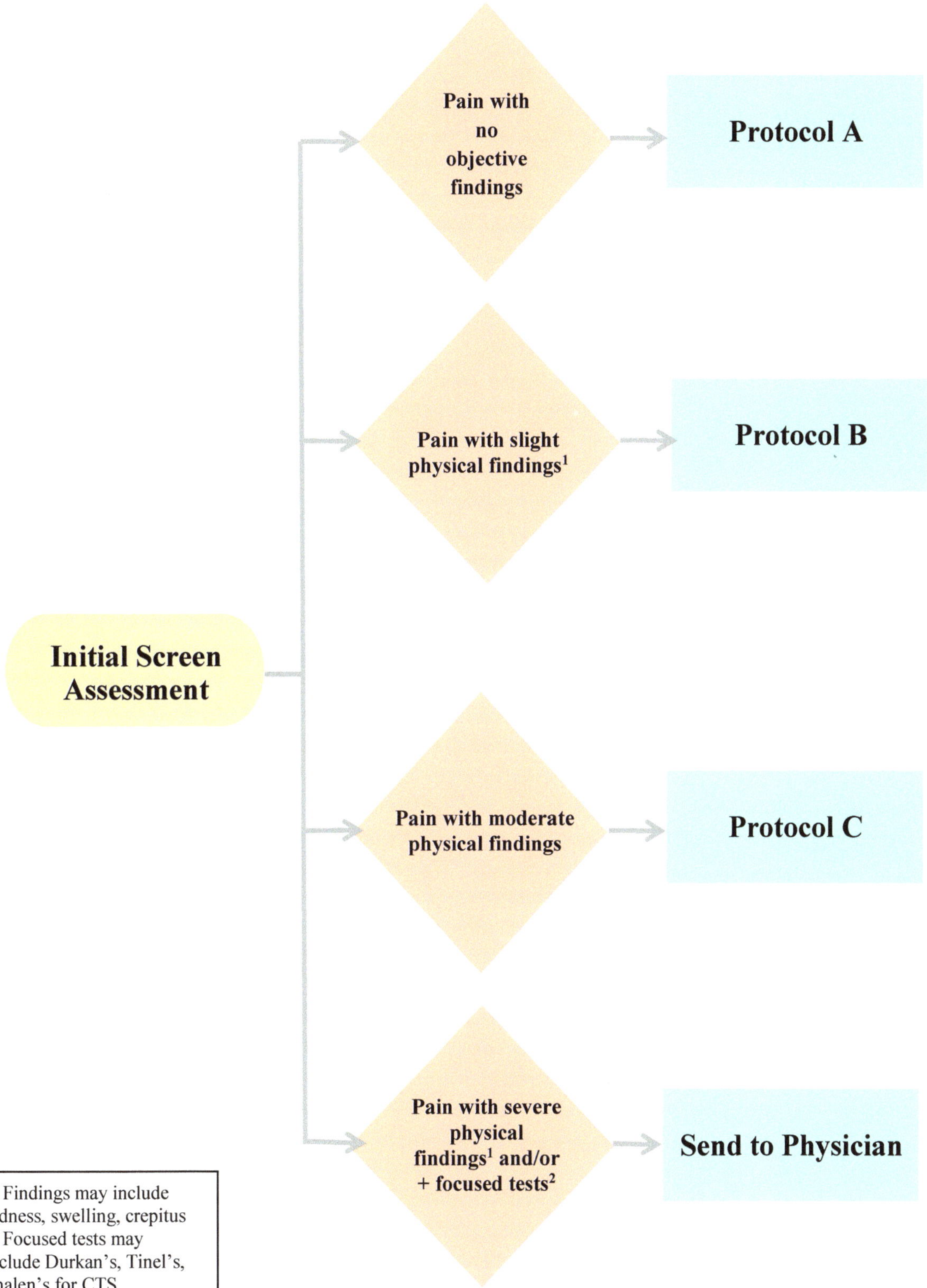

1. Findings may include redness, swelling, crepitus
2. Focused tests may include Durkan's, Tinel's, Phalen's for CTS, impingement tests for RTC, etc.

Treatment Pathways

There are three general treatment pathways germane to this CTS management protocol.

Treatment Pathway 1

- Ice[3]
- Medications[4]
- Regular job or job modification
- Stretching exercises[5]

Treatment Pathway 2

- Ice[3]
- Medications[4]
- Transition Duty

Treatment Pathway 3

- Ice[3]
- Medications[4]
- Transitional Duty
- Splints / Supports

3. 15 to 20 minutes per day, 3 times per day
4. Ibuprofen / Naproxen sodium / Ketoprofen / Aspirin or in the presence of gastric or duodenal ulcer or GERD, acetaminophen may be substituted. Do not use two or more NSAIDs together.
5. Stretching exercises are not indicated in the presence of acute pain.

Carpal Tunnel Syndrome: Evidence based research shows that the highest sensitivity for findings regarding CTS include a positive Katz hand diagram (the patient can trace on their hand or on paper the classic sensory distribution of numbness in the thumb, index, middle, and radial half of the ring finger) coupled with night time wakening and positive Flick symptomatology (where the patient frequently shakes their hand in order to get it to awaken from numbness). The best physical examination technique is the Durkan's compression test, which is superior to either the more traditional Phalen's or Tinel test.

Protocol A

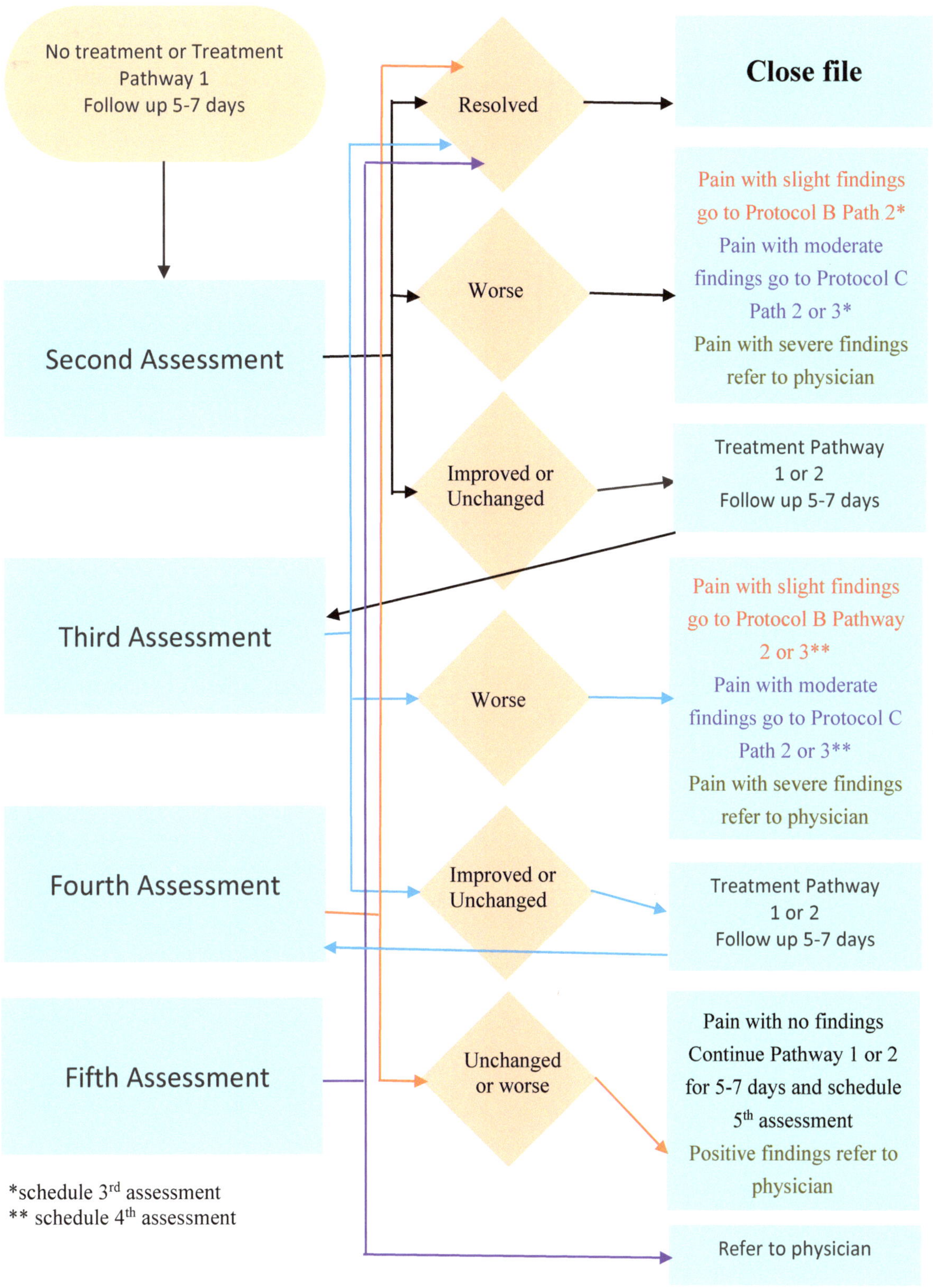

*schedule 3rd assessment
** schedule 4th assessment

Protocol B

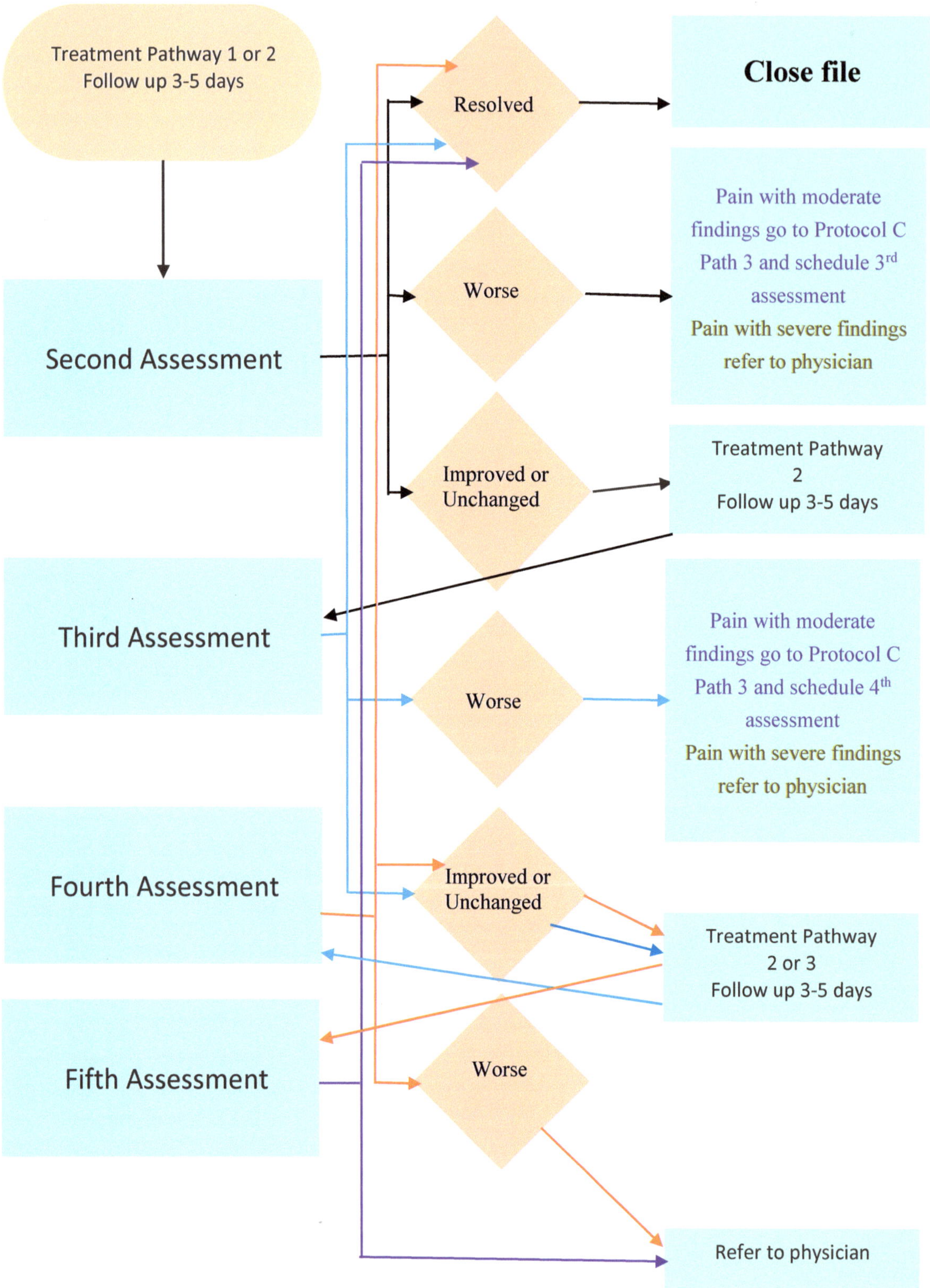

Treatment Pathway 1 or 2
Follow up 3-5 days
Resolved
Close file
Second Assessment
Worse
Pain with moderate findings go to Protocol C Path 3 and schedule 3rd assessment
Pain with severe findings refer to physician
Improved or Unchanged
Treatment Pathway 2
Follow up 3-5 days
Third Assessment
Worse
Pain with moderate findings go to Protocol C Path 3 and schedule 4th assessment
Pain with severe findings refer to physician
Fourth Assessment
Improved or Unchanged
Treatment Pathway 2 or 3
Follow up 3-5 days
Fifth Assessment
Worse
Refer to physician

Protocol C

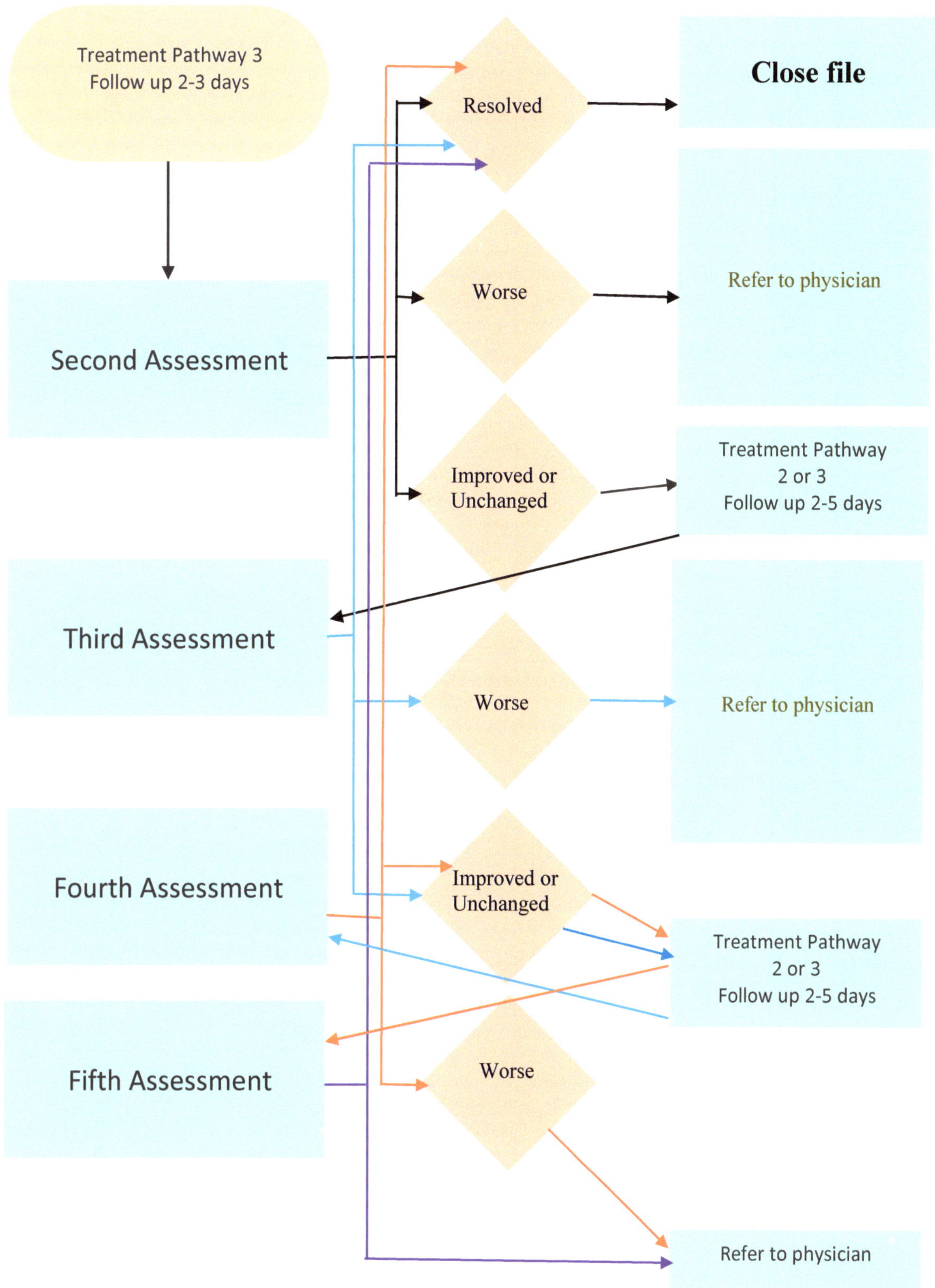

Treatment Pathway 3
Follow up 2-3 days
Second Assessment
Third Assessment
Fourth Assessment
Fifth Assessment
Resolved
Worse
Improved or Unchanged
Worse
Improved or Unchanged
Worse
Close file
Refer to physician
Treatment Pathway 2 or 3
Follow up 2-5 days
Refer to physician
Treatment Pathway 2 or 3
Follow up 2-5 days
Refer to physician

Notes:

Protocol A

If improved by not resolved, use conservative treatment pathway 1 and longer interval between assessments. If unchanged, use conservative treatment pathway 2 and shorter interval between assessments.

Protocol B

If improved but not resolved, use conservative treatment pathway 2 and longer interval between assessments. If unchanged, use conservative treatment pathway 3 and shorter intervals between assessments.

Protocol C

If improving but not resolved, potentially use conservative treatment pathway 2 and longer interval between assessments. If unchanged, use conservative treatment pathway 3 and shorter interval between assessments.

General

These protocols may be modified based upon the dynamics and specifics of workplace demands. For example, piece rate work or workers who are in a mandatory overtime situation may need to have more aggressive or frequent monitoring. Those workers who rotate among different job tasks may prove particularly challenging as there may be one task that is problematic while others pose no issues.

CTD NURSE ASSESSMENT

Company Name ____________________________ Date ____________________

Employee Information

Name: _____________________________________ SSN: ____________________

Job: ____ Time on job: ____________

Regular/Bid Job: _________Y ________N Additional Job: Y or N

Hand dominance: _______ Y ________N

- Date employee first noticed the problem: __________________________

- When was the current problem first reported to nurse/company? ___________

- What activities increase the problem?

  Excessive reach, push/pull, bending/stooping, pinching/gripping, pressure/force, twisting, vibration, unknown, other ________________________
  ____

- What factors does employee feel could have contributed to the problem?

  Lack of training, environmental temperature, tools/equipment, excessive job movements, length of time on job, hours on job (overtime), unable to keep knife sharp, unknown, other ____
  ____

- Any pre-existing medical treatment of:

  Diabetes, thyroid condition, arthritis, gastric or duodenal ulcer, currently pregnant, history of similar problem at this job or previous job

Notes / Definitions

Break-in period – Employees who are within their first six weeks of employment or in the first six weeks after a job transfer.

Slight symptoms – Symptoms which are mild in nature and for which there may not be any objective findings.

Moderate symptoms – Symptoms which indicate the presence of a detectable or potential problem.

Severe symptoms – Symptoms which indicate the need for physician intervention.

Applying cold – Ice is used to treat overuse strains and muscle/tendon disorders for relief of pain and swelling, thus allowing more mobility. Ice decreases the inflammation associated with CTD's even if no overt signs of inflammation (redness, warmth or swelling) are present. The use of ice may be inappropriate for Raynaud's disease (vibration syndrome), rheumatoid arthritis and diabetic conditions.

Non-steroid anti-inflammatory agents – These agents may be helpful in reducing inflammation and pain. Examples of these types of agents include aspirin, Ibuprofen/Advil, and Aleve/Naproxen.

Special exercise – If active exercises are utilized with employees with CTD's, they should be administered under the supervision of the Occupational Health nurse or physical therapist. If these active exercises are performed improperly, they may aggravate the existing condition.

Splints – A splint may be used to immobilize movement of the muscles, tendons and nerves. Splinting can result in a weakening of the muscle, loss of normal range of motion due to inactivity, or even greater stress on the area if activities are carried out while wearing the splint.

Job reassignment – A job reassignment must be chosen with knowledge of whether the new task will require the use of the injured tendons, or place pressure on the injured nerves. Inappropriate job reassignment can continue to injure the inflamed tendon or nerve, which can result in permanent symptoms or disability.

Restricted or light duty jobs are one of the most helpful treatments for CTD's. These jobs, if properly selected, allow the worker to perform while continuing to ensure recovery. Some CTD's require weeks (or months in rare cases) of reduced activity to allow for complete recovery.

*This outline was developed to provide guidelines to establish care and conformity in a medical management program. The majority of employees should improve with the medical management program. If a case does not resolve, the employee will be referred to a physician for care. The nurse can individualize the case using his/her discretion within the protocol guidelines.

Splints and Supports

There are a myriad of splints and supports available on the market today. As with many products, some are good and some not so good. The following guidelines are recommendations on splint usage that have been determined to be the most beneficial.

<u>**UPPER EXTREMITY**</u>

Finger Extension splints

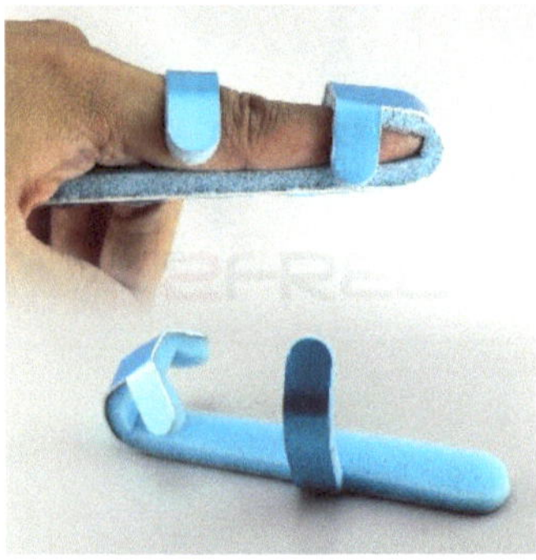

These splints are intended to be worn at night only for stenosing flexor tenosynovitis (trigger finger). It is best if these types of splints can be fashioned by a hand therapist. A temporary (several days) trial of a straight alumina foam-style splint may be utilized if hand therapy evaluation is not readily available.

Proflex or similar style wrist supports

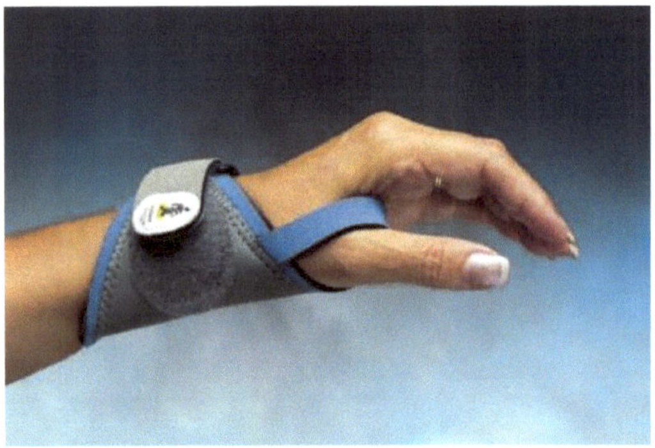

These splints are intended to be worn during the working hours. They are intended to hold the wrist in a neutral position without affecting the use of the fingers and thumb. Proper sizing is important. These splints are indicated for wrist flexor and extensor tendinitis and carpal tunnel syndrome.

Futuro or "cock-up" wrist splints

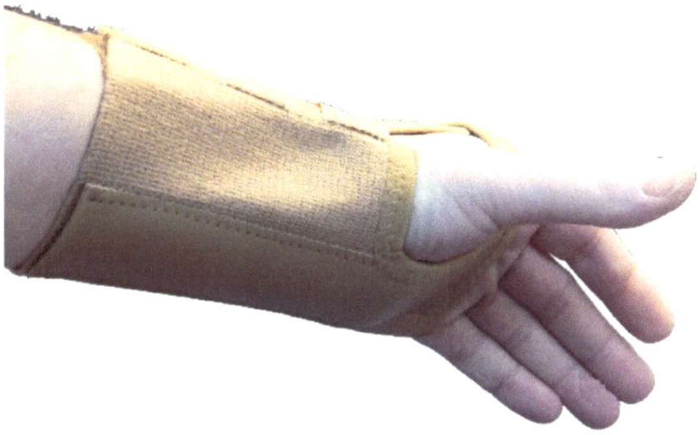

These splints are intended to be worn during sleep. They typically incorporate a metal stay on the flexor aspect of the splint. They are intended to keep the wrist in a neutral position while asleep, thereby relieving pressure on the wrist tendons and the carpal tunnel. Proper sizing is important. These splints are indicated for flexor and extensor tendinitis and carpal tunnel syndrome and are a second line treatment for tennis elbow.

Tennis elbow "counterforce" straps

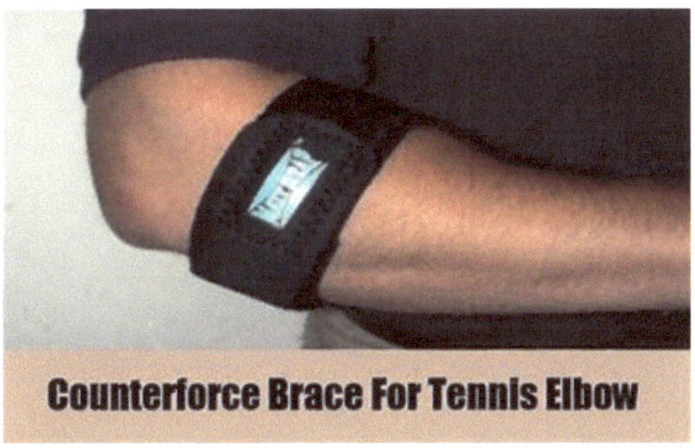

The tennis elbow strap is worn during working hours. It is worn to prevent transmission of force of the extensor muscle complex to the lateral epicondyle of the elbow. The tennis elbow strap should be non-elastic. There are many elastic versions available, which do not provide optimal decrease in the transmission of force over the muscle belly. The strap should be placed over the largest circumference of the proximal forearm, which is usually two fingerbreadths distal to the lateral epicondyle.

Thumb spica splints

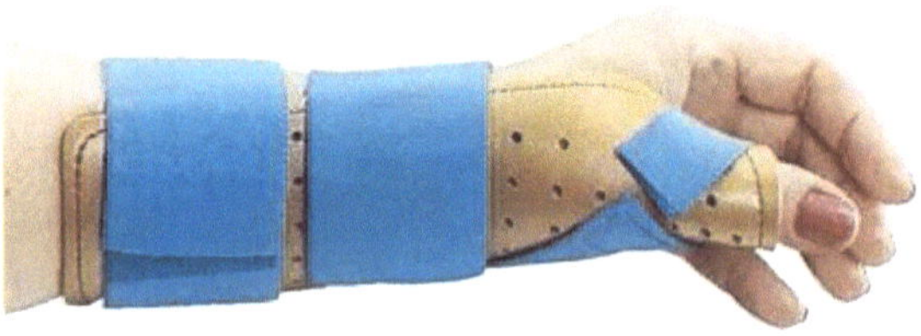

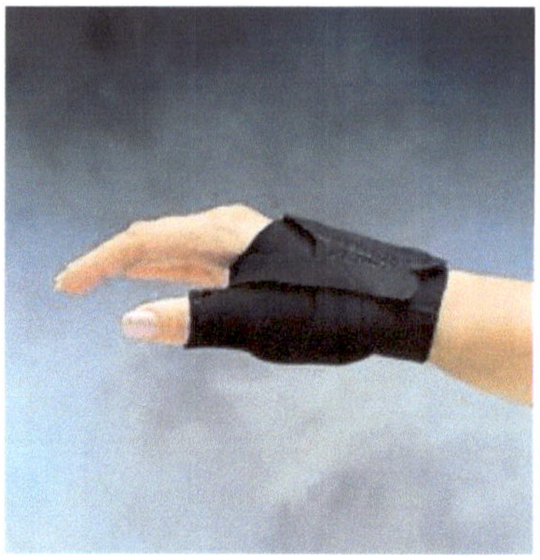

These splints are worn during the working hours. They are used in the treatment of de Quervain's tenosynovitis by immobilizing the CMC joint (and thereby the abductor pollicis longus and extensor pollicis brevis tendons). Proper sizing is important to eliminate over-constriction of the thumb. These splints range from the rigid (Freedom) to the non-rigid (Comfort Cool) variety.

LOWER EXTREMITY

Neoprene Knee Sleeves

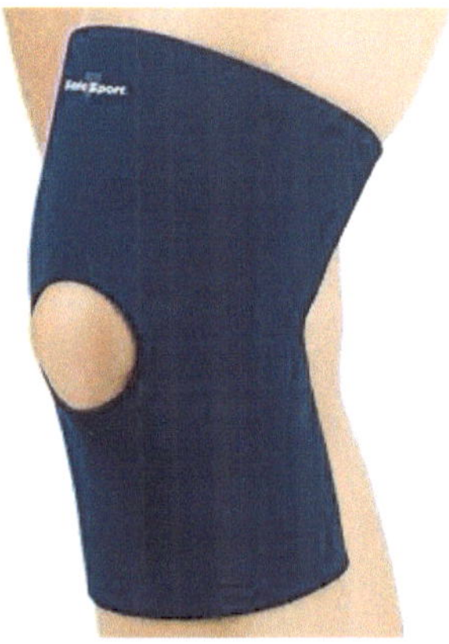

These slip-on knee supports are to be worn during the working hours. They can be used to treat many knee injuries and conditions including sprains, strains, bursitis, patellofemoral syndrome, and others. The open patella type is preferred (has a hole for the kneecap). Sizing is important, and you may determine that no one size is appropriate as individuals with large thigh-to-knee ratios may have difficulty.

Figure of Eight Ankle Supports

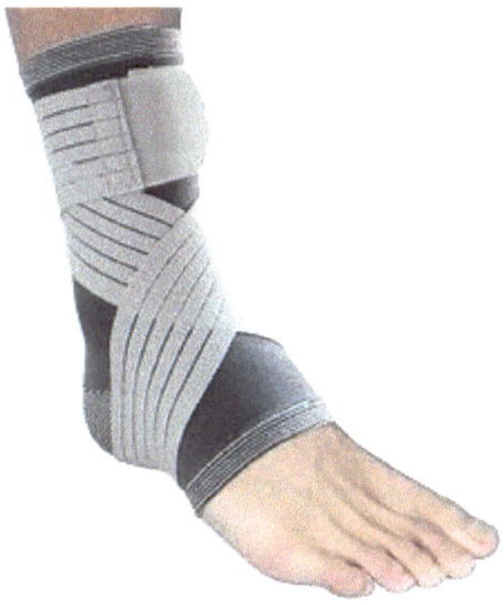

These supports slip on over the ankle and provide a combination of compression and support. They are used in the treatment of ankle sprains or strains. They are intended to be used only during the waking hours. They are not to be worn during sleep.

Heel Inserts (Wonderzorb or other)

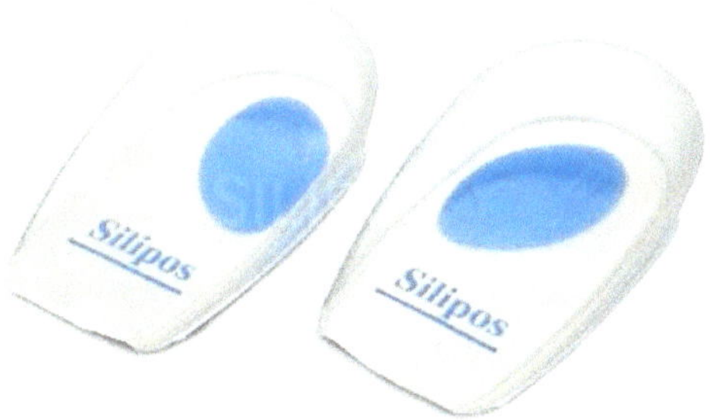

Heel inserts are used for temporary relief of pain from heel spurs or plantar fasciitis. It is important to understand that proper sizing, depending on the shoe style, is imperative.

Dorsi-wedge Nighttime Splint

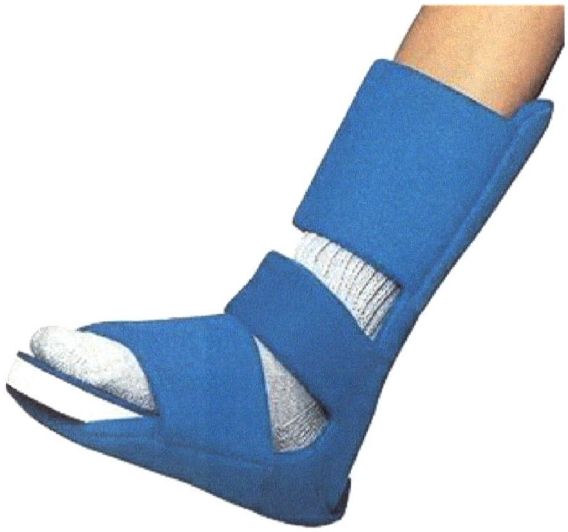

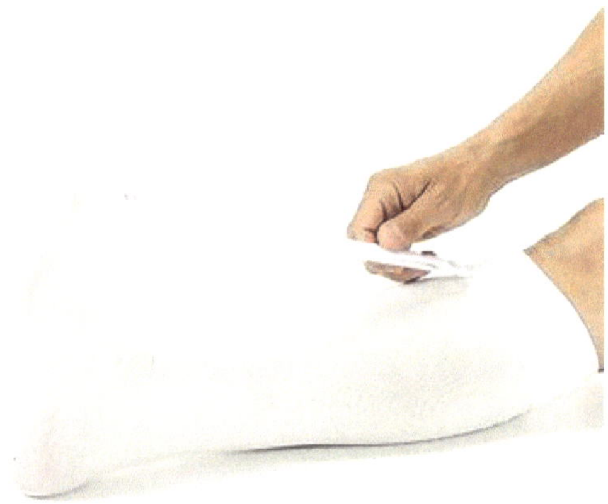

This splint is very similar to a rigid CAM walker set at 90 degrees, although lighter and is used for the treatment of plantar fasciitis. It is only worn while sleeping and is intended to stretch the plantar fascia so as to avoid the painful "first step in the morning" problem characteristic of plantar fasciitis. There is a non-rigid alternative to these splints called the Strassburg sock which accomplishes night time dorsiflexion, which may be used as an alternative if the rigid type splints are not tolerated.

Spenco (or similar) Arch Supports

Arch supports of this variety are used to help flat foot deformity (pes planus). Proper sizing is imperative.

SPINE

Lumbar Supports (Back Belts)

Clinical trials as published in the Journal of the American Medical Association support the conclusion that lumbar supports, commonly known as back belts, do not prevent injury and have no place in the treatment or prevention of low back pain. There are also numerous studies that support the fact that, with utilization of lumbar supports after a low back injury, the incidence of a subsequent low back injury with worsening outcomes is high.

There is only one reasonable situation in which use of a lumbar support may be medically justified, that being when it is used for abdominal support in individuals with extremely weak abdominal musculature support. This is a rare case. Therefore, on-site occupational nurses are precluded from issuing lumbar supports in the management or prevention of low back pain, unless specifically authorized by a physician specialist in occupational medicine.

Cervical Collars

Cervical collars are indicated only for severe and acute traumatic cervical spine injuries or as directed by a physician in a post-operative state. On-site occupational health nurses are not authorized to issue cervical collars for prevention or treatment of injuries, unless specifically authorized to do so by the occupational medicine physician, or by direction of emergency medical personnel in the transport of an employee who has sustained an acute traumatic cervical injury.

Steri-Strips (Butterfly Bandages)

Introduction:

Steri-strips can be used to:

1. Promote healing, or
2. In lieu of sutures.

It is very important to assess the wound to determine the need for sutures or if the use of steri-strips is indicated.

Mastisol® or similar liquid adhesive may be used with steri-strips to promote better adherence.

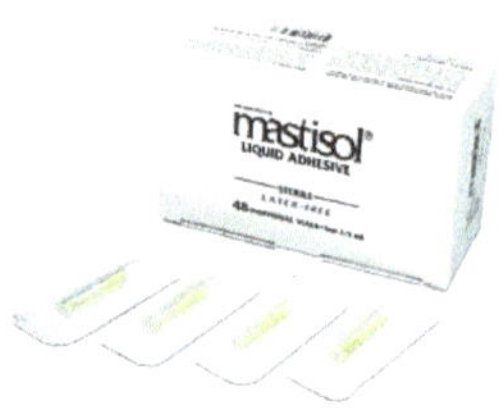

To Promote Healing:

1. May be used following suture removal to continue healing process.
2. ***Very*** superficial lacerations where underlying skin and structures are not involved.

In Lieu of Sutures:

1. Minor skin lacerations where underlying skin and structures, such as muscle, nerves or tendons are ***not*** involved, to approximate skin edges.

Treatment:

Refer to physician if:

1. Facial lacerations.
2. Over a joint or other area where steri-strips will not work.
3. If there is any doubt whether sutures are indicated.

Suicide

- If an employee threatens or confides that he/she is contemplating suicide, assist/refer employee to contact the local suicide crisis line or other similar agency.

  Suicide Crisis Line Phone: ____

  Other Agency: ____

  Other Agency Phone: ____

- ***Do not leave employee alone.*** Arrange for further assistance if you should have to leave.

- Provide assistance and support to employee as needed.

  - Follow-up with employee by phone or at next onsite visit.

Suture Removal

Introduction:

The Occupational Health nurse may remove sutures at the company site for lacerations under medical directives as listed.

Treatment:

1. Verify date for suture removal (check attending physician order).
2. Assess condition of suture site.
3. If site is healing well and does ***not*** appear infected (i.e., warmth, redness, painful movement, drainage), may use sterile suture removal set to remove sutures.
4. Sterile steri-strips may be used to further promote healing.
5. Apply clean dressing.
6. If site appears infected, or problems are noted with sutures, refer to attending physician.

Toothache

<u>Treatment</u>:

1. Advise employee to see dentist.
2. For temporary relief: acetaminophen (Tylenol®) 500 mg, 2 tabs PO every 4 hours.
3. See Appendix for other oral meds: Ibuprofen, ASA

Substance Abuse Testing

The Occupational Health nurse may be asked to provide onsite drug screening collection for a large number of companies.

Guidelines for specimen collection procedures follow the Department of Transportation (DOT) Testing Procedures as published in 49 CFR Part 40, amended on December 19, 2000. Although training and certification are not required for non-federal (non-regulated) collections, it is required for federal (regulated) tests, and it is recommended that any collector, regardless of type of collection, undergo training and proficiency testing as described in the federal guidelines.

The following pages outline steps that are to be followed in the collection procedure. For a complete discussion of the regulation, further details, please refer to the text of 49 CFR Part 40 and the SAMSHA Urine Specimen Collection Handbook. The web link for the collection handbook is:

http://www.workplace.samhsa.gov/DrugTesting/pdf/specimen_collection_handbook_2010_100908.pdf

Additionally, point of collection testing (POCT) has been gaining favor over recent years as the sensitivity and specificity of these "rapid test kits" becomes more standard. This presents a unique challenge to the occupational health nurse as they may be asked to now become not only a urine drug screen collector, but also an interpreter of these rapid tests. It is not possible to adequately describe all of the various different options for these tests that currently exist on the market. It is therefore suggested that if an employer wishes to choose this type of testing for their non-regulated program, that input is garnered from all stakeholders, including that of the occupational health nurse who could be conducting the test.

A resource that covers the general aspects of POCT testing can be found in this document from the American Association of Clinical Chemistry:

http://www.aacc.org/SiteCollectionDocuments/NACB/LMPG/POCT/Chapter%207.pdf

For non-regulated (non-Federal) drug testing, each individual state law addresses specifics. Please note that not every state follows the federal regulations, nor does every state have laws that address these issues to the same degree of specificity as federal law. Please direct any questions regarding non-federal employer drug testing to the corporate attorney.

An example of a state law is given here, for illustration purposes:

https://www.legis.iowa.gov/DOCS/ACO/IC/LINC/Section.730.5.pdf

Collection Procedure

The following steps describe a typical urine collection procedure under the Mandatory Guidelines:

STEPS

1. The collector prepares the collection site to collect urine specimens. All collection supplies must be available, the area properly secured, water sources secured, and bluing agent placed in all toilets.

Note: If access to a water supply in the restroom cannot be controlled, the collector may tell the donor that he or she will be listening at the entrance to the restroom for any sounds associated with the donor attempting to use the available sources of water. Alternatively, the collector may enter the restroom with the donor if the collector is the same gender as the donor but remains outside the toilet stall.

2. The collector begins the collection without delay after the donor arrives at the collection site.

Note: Do not wait because the donor is not ready, is unable to urinate, or an authorized employer or employee representative is delayed in arriving.

3. The collector requests the donor to present an acceptable form of identification as described in Chapter 5.

Note: If the donor cannot satisfy the identification requirement, the collector may proceed with the collection if the donor can provide <u>two</u> items of identification bearing his or her signature. After the donor signs the certification statement, the collector should compare the donor's signature with signatures on the identification that was presented. If the signatures match, the collector lists on the "Remarks" line the two items of identification used to identify the donor and states that "signature identification was confirmed." The collector then continues with the collection process. If the signature does not match the signatures on the two items of identification presented, the collector should state on the "Remarks" line that "signature identification is unconfirmed," discontinue the collection, and notify the collection site supervisor and the agency.

Note: In situations where the donor does not have either a photo identification or two other appropriate items of identification that could be used to verify identity and signature, this should not be automatically considered a refusal to test. The collector should proceed with the collection. The collector should provide sufficient information on the "Remarks" line to help the MRO and the agency make a determination regarding the validity of the specimen and the collection process.
Note: If the donor asks the collector to provide identification, the collector must show the donor some form of identification. It must include the collector's name and the employer's name, address, and telephone number. It does not have to be a picture identification or include a home address and telephone number.

4. The collector reviews the instructions on the back of the CCF with the donor.

5. The collector begins entering information and/or ensures that the required information is provided at the top of the CCF (the laboratory name and address and a pre-printed specimen ID number) and in Step 1 of the CCF (employer's name, address, and I.D. number (if applicable), MRO name, address, phone and fax number, donor SSN or employee ID number, reason for test, drug test to be performed, collection site information).

Note: A specific MRO's name and address must appear on the form rather than the name of the clinic or medical facility.

6. The collector asks the donor to remove any unnecessary outer clothing (e.g., coat, jacket, hat, etc.) and to leave any briefcase, purse, or other personal belongings he or she is carrying with the outer clothing. The donor may retain his or her wallet.

Note: The donor must not be asked to remove other articles of clothing, such as, shirts, pants, dresses, or under garments. Additionally, the donor must not be requested or required to remove all clothing and wear a hospital or examination gown.

7. The collector directs the donor to empty his or her pockets and display the items to ensure that no items are present that could be used to adulterate the specimen. If nothing is there that can be used to adulterate a specimen, the donor places the items back into the pockets and the collection procedure continues.

Note: If an item is found that appears to have been brought to the collection site with the intent to adulterate the specimen, a direct observed collection procedure is used. If the item appears to be inadvertently brought to the collection site, secure the item and continue with the normal collection procedure.

8. The collector instructs the donor to wash and dry his or her hands, preferably under the collector's observation and must not wash his or her hands again until after delivering the specimen to the collector.

Note: The donor must not be allowed any further access to water or other materials that could be used to adulterate/dilute the specimen.

9. The collector either gives the donor or allows the donor to select the collection container from the available supply. Either the collector or the donor, with both present, then unwraps or breaks the seal of the collection container.

Note: Do not unwrap or break the seal on any specimen bottle at this time.

Note: Do not allow the donor to take anything except the collection container into the room used for urination.

10. The collector directs the donor to go into the room used for urination, provide a specimen of at least 45 mL (split specimen collection) or 30 mL (single specimen collection), not to flush the toilet, and return with the specimen as soon as possible after completing the void.

Note: The donor is always permitted to provide a specimen in private unless a direct observed collection has been authorized.

Note: Pay close attention to the donor during the entire collection process to note any conduct that clearly indicates an attempt to substitute or adulterate a specimen. If you detect such conduct, immediately begin a new direct observed collection using a second CCF. Provide an appropriate comment on the "Remarks" line in Step 2 on the first CCF and submit it along with the specimen to the laboratory for testing. This will ensure that the laboratory knows that two separate specimens are being submitted for testing; the first one possibly being adulterated or substituted. Additionally, inform a supervisor that a collection took place under direct observation and the reason for doing so.

11. After the donor hands the specimen to the collector, the collector must measure the temperature of the specimen, check the specimen volume, and inspect the specimen for adulteration or substitution.

Temperature. Check the temperature of the specimen within four minutes after the donor hands you the specimen. The acceptable temperature range is 32E-38EC/ 90E-100EF. Temperature is determined by reading the temperature strip originally affixed to or placed on the outside of the collection container after the donor hands you the specimen.

A. If the temperature is within the acceptable range, the "Yes" box is marked in Step 2 on the CCF and the collector proceeds with the collection procedure.

B. If the temperature is outside the acceptable range, the "No" box is marked in Step 2 on the CCF and the collector immediately begins a direct observed collection procedure using a second CCF. The original specimen is sealed and sent with the first CCF to the laboratory with an appropriate comment on the "Remarks" line to indicate that a direct observed specimen was also being collected and submitted to the laboratory.

Specimen Volume. Check to make sure that the specimen contains a sufficient amount of urine (i.e., 30 mL for a single specimen collection, 45 mL for a split specimen collection).

A. Single specimen collection. If the volume is less than 30 mL, the action taken will depend on whether the temperature of the specimen is in or outside the acceptable range.

1. If the temperature is in the acceptable range, the specimen is discarded, and a second specimen is collected. The collector may use the same CCF for the second specimen but must use a new specimen collection container. If the donor fails for any reason to provide 30 mL of urine for the second specimen collected, the collector will contact the agency to obtain guidance on the action to be taken.

2. If the temperature is outside the acceptable range, a second specimen is collected under direct observation and both specimens are sent to the laboratory for testing. The collector must use a separate CCF for each specimen and provide an appropriate comment on each CCF to indicate why two specimens were collected. If the donor fails for any reason to provide 30 mL of urine for the

second specimen collected, the collector will contact the agency to obtain guidance on the action to be taken.

Note: In either case when a second specimen is to be collected, HHS permits giving the donor a reasonable amount of fluid to drink to provide a second specimen distributed reasonably through a period of up to 3 hours, or until the donor has provided a new sufficient amount of urine, whichever occurs first.

B. Split specimen collection. If the volume is less than 30 mL, the action taken will depend on whether the temperature of the specimen is in or outside the acceptable temperature range.

1. If the temperature is in the acceptable range, the specimen is discarded, and a second specimen is collected. The collector may use the original CCF for the second specimen but should use a new specimen collection container.
If the donor fails to provide 45 mL for the second specimen collected, the donor forfeits the right to the use of a split specimen collection procedure and the collector submits the second specimen as a single specimen collection with an appropriate comment on the "Remarks" line on the CCF.

2. If the temperature is outside the acceptable range, a second specimen is collected under direct observation and both specimens are sent to the laboratory for testing. The collector must use a separate CCF for each specimen and provide an appropriate comment on each CCF to indicate why two specimens were collected.

If the donor fails to provide 45 mL for the second specimen collected, the donor forfeits the right to the use of a split specimen collection procedure and the collector submits the second specimen as a single specimen collection (regardless of the volume collected) with an appropriate comment on the "Remarks" line on the CCF.

Note: In either case when a second specimen is to be collected, HHS permits giving the donor a reasonable amount of fluid to drink to provide a second specimen distributed reasonably through a period of up to 3 hours, or until the donor has provided a new sufficient amount of urine, whichever occurs first.

C. Split specimen collection. If the volume is between 30 and 45 mL, the action taken will depend on whether the temperature of the specimen is in or outside the acceptable temperature range.

1. If the temperature is in the acceptable range, all of the urine should be poured into one specimen bottle (Bottle A). Bottle A is sent to the laboratory along with the CCF. The collector should provide an appropriate comment on the "Remarks" line on the CCF that the donor did not provide a sufficient volume of urine for the split (Bottle B) specimen. The donor forfeits the use of a split specimen collection procedure.

2. If the temperature is <u>outside</u> the acceptable range, a second specimen is collected under direct observation and both specimens are sent to the laboratory for testing. The collector must use a separate CCF for each specimen and provide an appropriate comment on each CCF to indicate why two specimens were collected.

If the donor fails to provide 45 mL for the second collection, the second specimen is submitted as a single specimen collection and the collector should provide an appropriate comment on the "Remarks" line on the CCF that the donor did not provide a sufficient volume of urine for the split (Bottle B) specimen. The donor forfeits the use of a split specimen collection procedure.

Note: HHS permits giving the donor a reasonable amount of fluid to drink to provide a second specimen distributed reasonably through a period of up to 3 hours, or until the donor has provided a new sufficient amount of urine, whichever occurs first.

<u>Adulteration or Substitution</u>. Inspect the specimen for unusual color, presence of foreign objects or material, or other signs of adulteration (e.g., if you notice any unusual odor). If it is apparent from this inspection that the donor has adulterated or substituted the specimen (e.g., the specimen is blue, exhibits excessive foaming when shaken, has smell of bleach), a second collection using direct observation procedures is conducted. The first specimen and the specimen collected using direct observation are both sent to the laboratory for testing. The first specimen is always sent to the laboratory even though it may have had an insufficient volume for either a single or split specimen collection.

If the donor does not provide the required amount of urine for the second collection using direct observation, the collector submits the second specimen as a single specimen collection (regardless of the volume) and provides appropriate comments on the "Remarks" line on both CCFs.

Note: When a second specimen is to be collected, HHS permits giving the donor a reasonable amount of fluid to drink to provide a second specimen distributed reasonably through a period of up to 3 hours, or until the donor has provided a new sufficient amount of urine, whichever occurs first.

Note: Under no circumstance is the collector permitted to collect and add or combine urine from two separate voids.

12. The sealed specimen bottle is then unwrapped/opened in the donor's presence after the donor gives the specimen in the collection container to the collector. The collector or the donor may unwrap/open the specimen bottle.

Note: There will be two specimen bottles to be unwrapped/opened if a split specimen was collected.

Note: Both the collector and donor will maintain visual contact of the specimen until the label/seal is placed over the specimen bottle cap/lid.

13. The collector pours the specimen from the collection container into a specimen bottle, places the lid/cap on the bottle, and uses the "A" bottle tamper-evident label/seal. The "B" bottle label is discarded. If a split specimen collection procedure is used, the collector pours 30 mL of urine into a specimen bottle, places the lid/cap on the bottle and uses the "A" bottle label/seal. The collector then pours the remaining urine (at least 15 mL) into a second bottle, places the lid/cap on the bottle, and uses the "B" bottle label/seal.

Note: The tamper-evident label/seal must be placed over the lid/cap to ensure that the lid/cap cannot be removed without destroying the label/seal. The donor must be present to observe the sealing of the specimen bottle(s).

14. The collector writes the date on the tamper-evident label(s)/seal(s). The donor is requested to initial the tamper-evident label(s)/seal(s).

Note: Occasionally, the tamper-evident label/seal provided with the CCF will not properly adhere to the specimen bottle because of environmental conditions (e.g., moisture, temperature, specimen bottle material). When this occurs, the collector should still apply the tamper-evident label/seal provided with the CCF and then apply a second, separate tamper-evident seal to seal the specimen bottle. This second seal should be placed perpendicular to the CCF label/seal to avoid obscuring information on the CCF label/seal. This second seal must be initialed and dated by the collector and should be initialed by the donor (i.e., if the donor is still present when it is apparent that the CCF label/seal is not properly adhering to the specimen bottle; however, a label/seal may appear to adhere when initially placed on the bottle, but after several minutes the label/seal begins to lift off along the edges). The collector must also provide an appropriate comment on the "Remarks" line (CCF, Step 2) stating why the second seal was used.

Note: If while sealing and initialing the CCF label/seal the collector or donor accidentally breaks/damages the seal, the collector must apply a second, separate tamper-evident seal to seal the specimen bottle. This second seal should be placed perpendicular to the CCF label/seal to avoid obscuring information on the CCF label/seal. This second seal must be initialed and dated by the collector and initialed by the donor. The collector must also provide an appropriate comment on the "Remarks" line (CCF, Step 2) stating why the second seal was used.

Note: Since the specimen bottle is now sealed with tamper-evident tape and does not have to be under the donor's direct observation, the donor is allowed to wash his or her hands if he or she desires to do so.

15. The donor reads the certification statement on Copy 2 of the CCF (Step 5), signs and dates the certification statement, provides date of birth, printed name, and day and evening contact phone numbers.

Note: If the donor refuses to sign the form, the collector must make a notation on the "Remarks" line to that effect. Otherwise, without the collector's comment, a CCF without the donor's signature could result in a canceled test. The same procedure should be followed if the donor refuses to initial the label(s).

16. The collector completes the chain of custody on the CCF (Step 4) by printing his or her name, signing where indicated, recording the date and time of the collection, and indicating the specific name of the delivery service to whom the specimen bottle(s) are being released.

17. The collector removes Copy 5 from the CCF and gives it to the donor. The donor may now leave the collection site.

Note: At this time, the collector can tell the donor to list any prescription and over-the-counter medications he or she may have recently taken on the back of the donor copy (Copy 5) of the CCF, but not on any other copy. This information will help the donor remember what medications he or she may have taken if a positive result is reported by the laboratory to the MRO.

18. The collector places the specimen bottle(s) and Copy1 of the CCF inside the appropriate pouches of the leak-resistant plastic bag, seals the pouches, and initials and dates the seal.

19. The collector places the sealed plastic bag in an appropriate shipping container (e.g., express carrier mailer) and seals the shipping container as appropriate.

Note: If a collector is collecting several specimens within a short period of time, the sealed plastic bags may be placed into a single shipping container. The collector must maintain visual contact of the sealed plastic bags until all plastic bags are sealed in the single shipping container.

Note: The collector must ensure that each specimen is shipped to a laboratory as expeditiously as possible, the same day preferably.

20. The collector sends Copy 2 to the MRO and Copy 4 to the employer. Copy 3 is retained by the collector.

The collection procedure is now complete.

Physical Assessment

The Occupational Health nurse may have the responsibility of doing post-job offer physical assessments for a company.

Title I of the Americans with Disability Act of 1992 and the Americans with Disabilities Act Amendment Act (ADAAA) of 2008 address guidelines for employers to follow regarding medical examinations and inquiries of potential employees.

Some of the most important points for the onsite nurse to remember include:

1. Whether the person is able to perform a specific job with or without an accommodation.

2. Whether the person can perform the job without posing a "direct threat" to the health and safety of the person or others.

3. Medical files are confidential. Section VI (6.5) Confidentiality states that "Information from all medical examinations and inquiries must be kept apart from general personnel files as a separate, confidential medical record; available only under limited conditions specified in the ADA." (See Section 6.5)

The onsite nurses' responsibility is to obtain the objective/subjective data and record it. (The process is more important than the result of the assessment.)

If there are any concerns or questions regarding the process, it is suggested that the potential employee be referred to an occupational medicine physician for examination.

Tetanus Immunization Status

Introduction:

The need for administering tetanus immunization depends on the patient's previous immunization status and the tetanus prone nature of the wound. The CDC recommends that one booster dose of Tdap be administered instead of Td alone due to the increased concern of pertussis transmission.

The ACIP and CDC consider tetanus prophylaxis in wound management to be very important. For a comprehensive review of the recommendations, the ACIP report is located at the web address below:

https://www.cdc.gov/mmwr/preview/mmwrhtml/rr5517a1.htm#top

The occupational health nurse is encouraged to consult the CDC website frequently and to register for their email notifications so to keep up to date on any changes to these recommendations.

Treatment: (consent form must be signed)

1. Previously immunized individuals: Individuals with superficial wounds who have received basic tetanus immunization but have not had a tetanus booster during the past five years, should receive a booster immunization.

2. Individuals without active immunization against tetanus: All individuals with superficial wound(s) who have never received basic tetanus immunization should be referred to a physician for evaluation.

3. Individuals with partial immunization: When the patient has not received the recommended series of three immunizations for tetanus (for example only one or two documented immunizations) and the last dose was received more than ten years ago, a subsequent immunization should be administered IM for both tetanus prone and non-tetanus prone wounds.

4. Contraindications: The only contraindication to tetanus boosting in the wounded patient is a history of neurological or severe hypersensitivity reaction following a previous dose. Local side effects alone do not preclude continued use.

5. Active immunization for pregnant women is just as important as those who are not pregnant. Pregnancy is NOT a contraindication to receiving tetanus immunization. However, since the pertussis component of the Tdap vaccine poses certain risks, the pregnant worker who needs tetanus immunization should receive Td only in all situations.

6. See the following summary pages for additional information on the management of patients.

Tdap Summary

Purpose: To reduce morbidity and mortality from tetanus, diphtheria, and (where indicated) pertussis by vaccinating all adults who meet the criteria established by the Centers for Disease Control and Prevention's Advisory Committee on Immunization Practices.

Policy: Under these standing orders, eligible nurses may vaccinate adults who meet the criteria below.

Procedure

1. Identify adults in need of vaccination against tetanus, diphtheria, and (where indicated) pertussis based on the following criteria:

    a. lack of documentation of at least 3 doses of tetanus- and diphtheria-containing toxoids

    b. younger than age 65 years with no history of pertussis-containing vaccine given since age 10 years

    c. completion of a 3-dose primary series of tetanus- and diphtheria-containing toxoids with receipt of the last dose being 10 years ago or longer

    d. recent deep and dirty wound (e.g., contaminated with dirt, feces, saliva) and lack of evidence of having received tetanus toxoid-containing vaccine in the previous 5 years

2. Screen all patients for contraindications and precautions to tetanus and diphtheria toxoids (Td) and, if applicable, pertussis vaccine (Tdap):

    a. **Contraindications:**

    - Tdap is contraindicated for persons with a history of serious allergic reaction (i.e., anaphylaxis) to any component of the vaccine. Because of the importance of tetanus vaccination, persons with a history of anaphylaxis to components included in any Tdap or Td vaccines should be referred to an allergist to determine whether they have a specific allergy to tetanus toxoid and can safely receive tetanus toxoid (TT) vaccinations.

- Tdap is contraindicated for adults with a history of encephalopathy (e.g., coma or prolonged seizures) not attributable to an identifiable cause within 7 days of administration of a vaccine with pertussis components. This contraindication is for the pertussis components, and these persons should receive Td instead of Tdap.

b. **Precautions:**

- o history of Guillain-Barré syndrome within 6 weeks of previous dose of tetanus toxoid-containing vaccine
- o an unstable neurologic condition
- o moderate or severe acute illness with or without fever
    - Note: Use of Td or Tdap is not contraindicated in pregnancy. At the provider's discretion, either vaccine may be administered during the 2nd or 3rd trimester.

3. Provide all patients with a copy of the most current federal Vaccine Information Statement (VIS). You must document, in the patient's medical record or office log, the publication date of the VIS and the date it was given to the patient. Provide non-English speaking patients with a copy of the VIS in their native language, if available; these can be found at www.immunize.org/vis.

4. Administer 0.5 mL Td (or Tdap, if appropriate) vaccine intramuscularly (22–25g, 1–1½" needle) in the deltoid muscle.

5. Provide subsequent doses of Td (a one-time dose of Tdap may be substituted for Td if younger than 65 years) to adults as follows:

a. to complete the primary 3-dose schedule: observe a minimum interval of 4 weeks between the first and second doses, and 6 months between the second and third doses.

b. to boost after primary schedule is complete: observe a 10-year interval since previous dose of Td/Tdap; if protection against pertussis is needed, an interval of 5 years is recommended and intervals as short as 2 years or less can be observed for parents and caregivers of infants younger than age 12 months, healthcare workers having direct patient contact, and adults in a pertussis outbreak setting.

c. In pregnancy, when indicated, give Td or Tdap in 2nd or 3rd trimester. If not administered during pregnancy, give Tdap in immediate postpartum period.

6. Document each patient's vaccine administration information and follow up in the following places:

a. **Medical chart:** Record the date the vaccine was administered, the manufacturer and lot number, the vaccination site and route, and the name and title of the person administering the vaccine. If vaccine was not given, record the reason(s) for nonreceipt of the vaccine (e.g., medical contraindication, patient refusal).

b. **Personal immunization record card:** Record the date of vaccination and the name/location of the administering clinic.

7. Be prepared for management of a medical emergency related to the administration of vaccine by having a written emergency medical protocol available, as well as equipment and medications.

8. Report all adverse reactions to Td and Tdap vaccines to the federal Vaccine Adverse Event Reporting System (VAERS) at www.vaers.hhs.gov or (800) 822-7967. VAERS report forms are available at www.vaers.hhs.gov.

OCCUPATIONAL HEALTH SERVICES
TETANUS, DIPHTHERIA, PERTUSSIS (Tdap)
CONSENT FORM

Name: ____

Address: ____

City/State: ______________________ Home Telephone: __________

Age: _____ Sex: ______ Employer: _________________________

Have you received instruction regarding Tdap/Diphtheria, Tetanus and Pertussis vaccine? Yes No

Have you ever had a reaction to past Diphtheria, Tetanus or Pertussis vaccines? (DTP, DT or Td) Yes No

If yes, what type of reaction?

____

Are you pregnant? Yes No

Are you allergic to latex or any component of the vaccine? Yes No

I have read or have had explained to me information about Tdap/ Diphtheria, Tetanus and Pertussis vaccine. I have had a chance to ask questions which were answered to my satisfaction. I believe I understand the benefits and risks of the Tdap/Diphtheria, Tetanus and Pertussis vaccine and request that the vaccine be given to me or to the person for whom I am authorized to make this request.

Signature ___________________________ Date ___________

Witness ____________________________ Date ___________

Manufacturer _________________ Lot# __________ Site _______

Other Vaccinations / Immunizations

Introduction:

The on-site occupational health nurse will oftentimes be the point person for the administration of vaccinations and immunizations other than tetanus, based upon a company program. These vaccinations may be performed as a result of prophylaxis, or as a result of identification of risk due to an injury or an exposure.

There are many immunizations that may be appropriate in an industrial or occupational setting.

The following immunizations are authorized to be administered by the on-site occupational health nurse. This is not intended to be an all-encompassing list. Any questions should be directed to the medical director for clarification. In all circumstances, the package insert should be followed concerning the dosage and route of administration unless there is a specific physician order to deviate from the instructions within the package insert.

<u>Immunizations:</u>

1. Hepatitis A
2. Hepatitis B
3. Influenza
4. MMR
5. Pneumococcus
6. Meningococcus
7. Varicella

Allergy & Hormone Injections

In certain circumstances, the occupational on-site nurse may be asked to administer allergy or hormone injections. In each situation, a physician authorization and protocol must be obtained.

Allergy Injections:

1. It is recommended that a physician, nurse practitioner, or physician's assistant be present in the clinic.

2. Epinephrine 1:1000 must be on hand in case of anaphylactic reaction. Initial dose is 0.3 to 0.5 ml.

3. Have client obtain records and physician order. Confirm name, mix, concentration, amount and site of administration.

4. Match serum with records and physician order. Confirm all details.

5. Roll vial of serum gently between palms to mix (do not shake).

6. Clean rubber top of vial with alcohol swab.

7. Use sterile allergy or TB syringe with a 26g needle to draw up ordered amount of serum.

8. Give client tissue or cotton ball to dab at injection site.

9. Instruct client to not scratch or rub the area.

10. Have the client wait 15-20 minutes, then re-check the injection site for local reactions.

11. Tell client when to return for next injection.

12. Document date, concentration, amount, site, and any adverse reactions.

Hormone injections:

Hormone injections may include but are not limited to: testosterone, estrogen, progesterone, erythropoietin, or growth hormone.

1. Obtain physician authorization for administration
2. Follow administration guidelines per package insert
3. Document administration date, amount, type of injection, site, and any adverse reactions.
4. Contact physician or medical director with questions.

Phlebotomy Authorization

On-site occupational health nurses are oftentimes asked to assist in health or risk screening activities sponsored by companies or sponsored by other organizations that are held on company premises. Additionally, they may be asked to assist in surveillance programs where periodic laboratory analysis is required.

If the on-site nurse has undergone the appropriate training for the performance of blood draws and/or finger stick determinations, they are authorized to do so under these directives.

The occupational health nurse may refer to their local hospital for any phlebotomy resources and to follow any example guidelines for procedural and protocol manners. Another excellent resource for best practices and standards is provided at this web address:

https://www.ephlebotomytraining.com/phlebotomy-procedure

If there any questions, please contact the medical director.

List of Approved Medications for On-site Use

1. Epinephrine – 0.3 to 0.5 ml of 1:1000 solution SC or IM for anaphylactic or asthmatic reaction. EpiPen or EpiPen Jr. according to weight of person.
2. Ibuprofen 200 mg tablets. Used for a variety of complaints. Dosage per specific directive.
3. Hydrocortisone cream or ointment 0.5 to 1.0%. Used primarily for dermatitis. See dermatitis protocol.
4. Triple antibiotic ointment. See specific protocol.
5. Bactroban. See burn directive
6. Bacitracin. See burn directive.
7. Silvadene cream. See burn directive.
8. Oxygen. See specific directive.
9. Benadryl (diphenhydramine) 25 mg tablets every 4-6 hours prn.
10. Sudafed (pseudoephedrine) 60 mg tablets every 4-6 hours prn.
11. Phenylephrine 10 mg tablets every 4 hours prn
12. Menthol gel prep. See specific protocol.
13. Waterjel Burn gel. See burn protocol.
14. Acetaminophen tablets 325 mg or 500 mg tablets. Used for a variety of purposes. See specific protocol.
15. Naproxen sodium 220 mg tablets. Used for a variety of complaints. Dosage per specific directive
16. Ketoprofen 12.5 mg tablets. Used for a variety of complaints. Dosage per specific directive.
17. Aloe Vera gel. Used for a variety of skin complaints.
18. Lamisil AT for fungal dermatitis.

19. Lotrimin AF for fungal dermatitis.
20. Tinactin for fungal dermatitis.
21. Kerodex for skin protection.
22. Skin ProTec for skin protection.
23. ASA (aspirin) 325 mg. Dosage per directive.
24. ____
25. ____
26. ____
27. ____
28. ____
29. ____
30. ____

Medication Fact Listings

Acetaminophen

1. Acts as an:
    a. anti-pyretic
    b. analgesic
2. Does NOT
    a. have anti-inflammatory properties
    b. Carry risk for gastrointestinal bleeding
3. Maximum adult dose is 4,000 mg per 24 hours
4. Is safe in pregnancy
5. Is safe if breastfeeding
6. Potential drug interactions:
    a. Alcohol
    b. Barbiturates
    c. Dilantin
    d. Tegretol

Aspirin

1. Acts as an:
    a. Anti-pyretic
    b. Anti-inflammatory
    c. Analgesic
2. Do NOT use if patients:
    a. Are sensitive to non-steroidal drugs (NSAIDs)
    b. Have a history of bleeding ulcer
    c. Are less than 18 years of age
    d. Are less than one week from a scheduled surgery
3. Maximum dosage is 4000 mg in 24 hours
4. Do NOT use in pregnancy
5. Do NOT use if breastfeeding
6. Drug interactions and contraindications:
    a. Do NOT use if taking other anti-inflammatories
    b. Do NOT use if taking blood thinners unless authorized by physician
    c. Use of alcohol increases risk of gastrointestinal bleeding

Ibuprofen

1. Acts as an:
    a. Anti-pyretic
    b. Anti-inflammatory
    c. Analgesic
2. Do NOT use if:
    a. Aspirin allergy or asthma like reactions to taking aspirin
    b. Previous reaction to NSAIDs
    c. Patient taking blood thinners without doctor authorization
3. Do NOT use in pregnancy
4. Do NOT use if breastfeeding
5. Be cautious in patients with:
    a. Hypertension
    b. Previous ulcer history
    c. Prior photosensitivity reaction to any medication
6. Drug interactions with:
    a. Digoxin
    b. Dilantin
    c. Lithium
    d. Loop diuretics
    e. Aspirin
7. Common side effects:
    a. Nausea and vomiting
    b. Diarrhea
    c. Rash
    d. Flatulence
8. General on-site limitations are no greater than 3 days continuous use for either fever or pain without physician evaluation.

Blood Profile / Laboratory Information

Regular blood testing is one of the most important ways to keep track of overall physical well-being. Getting tested at routine intervals can allow the ability to track changes over time and empower your health care provides to make informed decisions about your health.

Often, the occupational health nurse is involved in employee health screens or wellness activities. This section is intended to provide a general overview of the common laboratory screening tests and how they can be used.

1. Complete blood count

A routine complete blood count (CBC) test checks for levels of 10 different components of every major cell in your blood: white blood cells, red blood cells, and platelets. Important components measured by this test include red blood cell count, hemoglobin, and hematocrit.
Here's the typical range of results:

Component	Normal range
red blood cells	**men:** 4.32–5.72 million cells/mcL; **women:** 3.90–5.03 million cells/mcL
white blood cells	3,500 to 10,500 cells/mcL
platelets	150,000 to 450,000/mcL
hemoglobin	**men:** 13.5–17.5 grams/deciliter (g/dL); **women:** 12.0–15.5 g/dL
hematocrit	**men:** 38.8–50.0 percent; **women:** 34.9–44.5 percent

Abnormal levels of these components may indicate:

- nutritional deficiencies, such as vitamin B-6 or B-12
- iron deficiency
- bone marrow issues
- tissue inflammation

- infection
- heart conditions
- cancer

2. Basic metabolic panel

A basic metabolic panel (BMP) checks for levels of certain compounds in the blood, such as:

- electrolytes
- calcium
- glucose
- sodium
- potassium
- carbon dioxide
- chloride
- blood urea nitrogen (BUN)
- creatinine
-

This test requires you to fast for at least eight hours before your blood is drawn.

Normal ranges will vary slightly for adults over the age of 60 years.

Test	Normal range (adults 18-60 years old)	Normal range (adults over 60 years old)	Category
BUN (blood urea nitrogen)	6-20 mg/dL (milligrams per deciliter of blood)	8-23 mg/dL	kidney test
creatinine	0.9-1.3 mg/dL for men; 0.6-1.1 mg/dL for women	0.8-1.3 mg/dL for men; 0.6-1.2 mg/dL for women	kidney test
glucose	70-99 mg/dL	70-99 mg/dL	sugar metabolism
albumin	3.4-5.4 g/dL (grams per deciliter of blood)	3.4-5.4 g/dL	blood protein

CO_2 (carbon dioxide or bicarbonate)	23-29 mEq/L (milliequivalent units per liter of blood)	23-31 mEq/L (adults 61-90 years old); 20-29 mEq/L (adults over 90 years old)	electrolyte panel
Ca+ (calcium)	8.6-10.2 mg/dL	8.6-10.2 mg/dL	electrolyte panel
Na+ (sodium)	136-145 mEq/L	132-146 mEq/L (adults over 90 years old)	electrolyte panel
K+ (potassium)	3.5-5.1 mEq/L	3.5-5.1 mEq/L	electrolyte panel
Cl- (chloride)	98-107 mEq/L	98-111 mEq/L (adults over 90 years old)	electrolyte panel

Abnormal results may indicate kidney disease, diabetes, or hormone imbalances. Your doctor will perform follow-up tests to diagnose any of these conditions.

3. Complete metabolic panel

A complete metabolic panel (CMP) includes all the measurements of a BMP as well as additional proteins and substances related to liver function:

- albumin
- total protein
- alkaline phosphatase (ALP)
- alanine aminotransferase (ALT)
- aspartate aminotransferase (AST)
- bilirubin

The same conclusions can be drawn from a CMP as from a BMP for the same substances that a BMP covers. Other abnormal levels can also indicate underlying conditions, such as:

High levels	Low levels

ALP	• bile duct blockage • cirrhosis • gallbladder inflammation • gallstones • hepatitis • Paget's disease	• bone metabolism disorders • heart surgery • malnourishment • zinc deficiency
ALT	• cirrhosis • hepatitis • liver cancer • liver damage	considered normal
AST	• cirrhosis • heart conditions • hepatitis • mononucleosis • (mono)pancreatitis	considered normal
Bilirubin	• abnormal red blood cell destruction (hemolysis) • adverse medication reactions • bile duct blockage • Gilbert's syndrome • hepatitis	not a concern

4. Lipid panel

This test checks levels of two types of cholesterol:

- high-density lipoprotein (HDL), or "good" cholesterol
- low-density lipoprotein (LDL), or "bad" cholesterol

HDL is "good" because it removes harmful substances from your blood and helps the liver break them down into waste. LDL is "bad" because it can cause plaque to develop in your arteries, increasing your risk of heart disease.

You need to fast for at least 8 hours before this test.
Here are the ranges for each type:

	High	Low
HDL	> 60 mg/dL	**men:** < 40 mg/dL; **women:** < 50 mg/dL
LDL	> 160 mg/dL	< 100 mg/dL

Normal levels can also vary by age.

5. Thyroid panel

A thyroid panel, or thyroid function test, checks how well your thyroid is producing and reacting to certain hormones, such as:

- **Triiodothyronine (T3).** Along with T4, this regulates your heart rate and body temperature.
- **T3 resin uptake (RU).** This measures how well a hormone called thyroxin-binding globulin is binding.
- **Thyroxine (T4).** Along with T3, this regulates your metabolism and how you grow.
- **Thyroid-stimulating hormone (TSH).** This helps regulate the levels of hormones your thyroid releases.

Your thyroid, a tiny gland in your neck, helps regulate bodily functions like your mood, energy level, and overall metabolism.

Here are normal results:

- **T3:** 100–200 nanograms per deciliter of blood (ng/dL)
- **T3RU:** depends on T3 levels (low if T3 levels are high, and vice versa)
- **T4:** 5.0–12.0 micrograms per deciliter (μg/dL)
- **TSH:** 0.4–4.0 milli-international units per liter of blood (mIU/L)

Abnormal levels of these hormones can indicate numerous conditions, such as low protein levels, thyroid growth disorders, and abnormal levels of testosterone or estrogen.

6. Enzyme markers

Enzymes are proteins that help your body accomplish certain chemical processes, such as breaking down food and clotting blood. They're used throughout your body for many vital functions. Abnormal enzyme levels can indicate many different conditions.

Common enzymes tested include:

- **Creatine phosphokinase (CPK-1).** This is found in your lungs and brain. High levels can indicate brain injuries or cancer.
- **CPK-2 (CK-MB).** These enzymes are found in your heart. They often increase in your blood after a heart attack or other heart injury.
- **CPK-3.** These enzymes are also found in your heart. They often result from muscle inflammation, injury, or intense exercise.
- **Troponin.** This is a heart enzyme that can leak into your blood and results from heart injury.

Here are the normal ranges for the enzyme listed above:

- **CPK-1:** about 200 units per liter (U/L)
- **CPK-2:** 5–25 international units per liter (IU/L)
- **CPK-3:** about 200 U/L
- **troponin:** < 0.02 ng/mL

7. Sexually transmitted disease tests

Many sexually transmitted diseases (STDs) can be diagnosed using a blood sample. These tests are often combined with urine samples or swabs of infected tissue for more accurate diagnoses.

The following STDs can be diagnosed with blood tests:

- chlamydia
- gonorrhea
- herpes
- HIV
- Syphilis

Blood tests aren't always accurate right after contracting an infection. For an HIV infection, for example, you may need to wait at least a month before a blood test can detect the virus.

8. Coagulation panel

Coagulation tests measure how well your blood clots and how long it takes for your blood to clot. Examples include the prothrombin time (PT) test and fibrinogen activity test.

Clotting is a crucial process that helps your stop bleeding after a cut or wound. But a clot in a vein or artery can be deadly, blocking blood flow to your brain, heart, or lungs and causing heart attack or strokes.

Coagulation test results vary based on your health and any underlying conditions that may affect clotting.

Results from this test can be used to diagnose:

- acute myeloid leukemia
- excessive bleeding (hemophilia)
- thrombosis
- liver conditions
- vitamin K deficiency

9. DHEA-sulfate serum test

The dehydroepiandrosterone (DHEA) hormone comes from your adrenal glands. This test measures whether it's too high or too low.

In men, DHEA helps develop traits like body hair growth, so low levels are considered abnormal. In women, high levels can cause typically male traits, like excess body hair, to develop, so low levels are normal.

Low levels in men are called DHEA deficiency, which can be caused by:

- type 2 diabetes
- kidney disease
- anorexia nervosa
- AIDS

High levels in men or women can result from:

- cancer or tumor in adrenal glands
- early onset of puberty from congenital adrenal hyperplasia
- abnormal genital development
- polycystic ovary syndrome (in women)

10. C-reactive protein test

C-reactive protein (CRP) is made by your liver when tissues in your body are inflamed. High CRP levels indicate inflammation from a variety of causes, including:

- artery inflammation
- infection
- inflammatory bowel disease (IBD)
- heart disease
- rheumatoid arthritis
- lupus
- cancer

The higher the level in your results, the higher your risk of heart disease:

- **< 1 mg/L:** low risk
- **1–2.9 mg/L:** intermediate risk
- **> 3 mg/L:** high risk
- **> 10 mg/L:** extremely high risk, and further testing should be done to diagnose high levels of inflammation in your body

Protocol for Movement

Movement of the Injured Worker

Minor:

In cases of minor injury or illness, where the employee is stabilized onsite (controlled bleeding, fatiness, contusions), the first aider has several alternatives:

1. Minor first aid treatment with follow-up report to Occupational Health Nurse.
2. For personal injury or illness, have employee contact personal physician
3. For work-related illness or injury, have supervisor contact physician
4. Contact family to take to physician
5. Contact supervisor to arrange transportation to hospital or physician
6. Contact Occupational Health Clinic for advice

Major:

Sever injury or illness (uncontrolled bleeding, shock, respiratory difficulties, industrial accidents) necessitate emergency treatment. As the employee is being stabilized onsite, the first aider should:

1. Direct an individual to contact ambulance for immediate transfer
2. Contact Company Coordinator or supervisor who should:
    a) Contact family
    b) Contact occupational health clinic to facilitate hospital arrangements
    c) Contact appropriate Company department
3. Accompany employee until he/she is safely in hands of emergency medical services team

Tuberculosis Infection Control Plan

This document makes recommendations for reducing the risk of transmitting M. tuberculosis (TB) to employees, healthcare workers (HCWs), visitors, and others.

Introduction to Tuberculosis

Tuberculosis (TB) is a disease caused by a bacterium, Mycobacterium tuberculosis. TB is spread primarily by airborne droplets coughed up from the lungs of persons with active disease. Once inhaled, the organisms establish infection in the lungs and then disseminate throughout the body before the immune response brings the primary infection under control. Most infected persons have no symptoms of disease. Following infection, a small percentage of individuals will develop symptoms. About ten percent of persons who become infected will develop an active case of TB during their lifetimes.

The risk of developing active disease is enhanced by a number of factors, including HIV infection, pharmacologic immuno-suppression (steroids), underlying medical conditions such as diabetes mellitus and sudden weight loss.

For decades the prevalence of tuberculosis in the United States was declining. Since the mid 1980's, however, the number of tuberculosis cases increased. This increase appears to be fueled by the development of the epidemic of HIV infection in this country. Those areas seeing the largest caseloads of HIV infection are the same areas experiencing the largest increases in tuberculosis cases. In 1992 pulmonary tuberculosis was made an AIDS-defining illness. In 1993 the number of cases of tuberculosis in this country decreased from the previous year. This decline may be due to reporting of tuberculosis cases as AIDS-defining illnesses, rather than reporting through tuberculosis control channels or to greater success in having patients complete a course of treatment.

Risk Assessment

With the increased prevalence of tuberculosis in the United States, it is important to realize that the disease is spread almost exclusively from individuals who have pulmonary infection and who cough infectious organisms into the air which may be inhaled by others. Rarely, a person with a soft tissue tuberculosis infection may spread organisms through aerosols from drainage at their infected site. Workers in front line positions may encounter tuberculosis among individuals who have not yet been diagnosed. Personnel with contact should be aware of this problem. Laboratory personnel who handle the organism, M. tuberculosis, may also be at risk. An ongoing employee tuberculin screening program is available to monitor workers who may be at risk of becoming occupationally infected with tuberculosis.

Tuberculosis Control Measures

Tuberculosis control involves a hierarchy of interventions. Those interventions are:

1) administrative controls

2) source control

3) engineering controls

4) personal protective equipment.

Administrative Controls

Administrative controls include the education of staff and development of policies and practices for the rapid identification and isolation of individuals suspect of having tuberculosis.

Tuberculosis Guidelines: Management of Individuals to Prevent Tuberculosis Exposures

1. Rapid identification, isolation of the patient and initiation of treatment is the best way to control tuberculosis and prevent its spread.

2. Professional staff should be aware of the presence of a cough. Any individual complaining of a cough should be questioned regarding symptoms and risk factors for tuberculosis. Any individual suspected of having tuberculosis based on symptoms described or on the basis of chest x-ray findings should be immediately given a mask to wear. The employee should be referred to their personal healthcare provider for more careful evaluation as soon as possible.

3. If an individual has a productive cough of more than two weeks duration a mask should be placed on the patient. Patients at particular risk of tuberculosis include those on immuno-suppressive medications (e.g. cyclosporine, steroids), HIV infected persons, persons born in countries with high endemic rates of TB, alcoholics and those with kidney failure, pulmonary disease and other conditions.

4. If cough is not identified by questioning or evaluation proceed with appropriate work-up for patient.

Source Control

Source control is a very important aspect of tuberculosis control. The "source" is the coughing patient with active pulmonary or laryngeal tuberculosis. The ultimate means of source control is to have a patient with active tuberculosis successfully complete a course of therapy. It is now recommended that all patients with tuberculosis receive directly observed therapy, which involves the observed administration of all a patient's medication. Factors such as homelessness, substance abuse, psychiatric disorders, as well as other problems may impair the patient's ability to complete therapy. Attempts should be made to identify factors which may interfere with a patient's ability to take proper medication. While waiting for anti-tuberculosis therapy to take effect, the source control can be affected by having a patient wear a mask or simply cover his/her mouth while coughing. The mask may be a paper surgical mask. Patients known or suspected to have tuberculosis should be restricted in their workplace as determined by an occupational medicine physician.

Engineering Controls

Engineering controls are utilized to decontaminate the air in high-risk areas.

Respiratory Protection

The last line of defense against the spread of tuberculosis is the use of personal protective equipment. Respiratory devices are employed to prevent the inhalation of infectious droplets. They will be used in situations where the patient has not yet received sufficient treatment to be rendered non-infectious and when environmental controls may not provide adequate protection. Appropriate respiratory protection will be provided to staff who are at-risk at no cost. Before wearing a respirator, personnel must be evaluated and instructed in respirator selection, fit testing, and use.

What to do in the event of an exposure

If an employee has been exposed to tuberculosis in the course of his/her duties, the employee should report this to the immediate supervisor for possible tuberculosis screening. The Local Health Department will assist in investigating occupational exposures to tuberculosis to determine if there have been any unprotected exposures. In instances of unprotected exposure, the exposed individuals are identified and are instructed where to report for testing. Individuals who become infected with tuberculosis (develop a positive skin test reaction) following an exposure are not able to transmit tuberculosis unless they develop an active case of TB.

Screening of employees for tuberculosis

A Mantoux PPD intradermal skin test or the interferon gamma release assay (IGRA) test shall be administered at the time of the post-job offer physical examination. Every employee who is at-risk of occupational exposure to tuberculosis must be screened on an annual basis. Persons working in high exposure areas or occupations should be screened twice yearly.

The program of tuberculin screening is administered by the Safety Director and/or Occupational Health Nurse. The screening protocol used is attached (see Appendix A). Should an employee be found to have a positive test for tuberculosis further evaluation would be necessary, including, if needed, a chest radiograph. If the screening test is positive, preventive medicine may be indicated to reduce the risk of developing active disease. A decision whether to take that medicine should be made in conjunction with advice provided by the Local Health Department and the employee's personal physician. Standard guidelines from the American Thoracic Society are employed in the decision to recommend prophylaxis following tuberculosis infection.

Individual Responsibilities
Responsibilities of Company:

1) Prompt referral of patients suspected or proven to have active pulmonary tuberculosis.

2) Notification of the Local Health Department of potential exposure of employees to tuberculosis.

Responsibilities of Safety Director and/or Occupational Health Nurse:

1) Training personnel who may be at-risk of occupational exposure to tuberculosis.

2) Training and fit-testing of personnel who may require respiratory protection.

3) Ensuring appropriate referral of employees suspected of having occupational exposure to a patient with active pulmonary tuberculosis or when an unsuspected tuberculosis exposure episode has occurred.

4) Development of "contact" lists when an exposure episode has occurred, so that appropriate screening maybe performed.

5) Periodic screening of at-risk employees for tuberculosis.

6) Screening of personnel following an unsuspected tuberculosis exposure episode.

7) Maintenance of centralized medical records allowing employee tracking.

Contacts for Information

Contact the County Health Department for more information on tuberculosis control.

Appendix A
Screening for TB Infection - Procedures

Screening for TB Infection

All employees be screened upon employment with an IGRA test. Multiple puncture tests are not recommended. After initial screening, TB screening tests should be repeated at least annually for all who are at risk of occupational exposure. Results of these tests should be compared with previous testing and with infection rates of the general population. More frequent screening should take place if there is an increase in:

- the incidence of either TB or HIV/AIDS; or

- the incidence of TB infection (positive tuberculin skin test reactions).

TB Skin Testing

The Mantoux tuberculin skin test is no longer the primary screening test of choice. The incident rate of incorrectly applied and incorrectly interpreted tests, along with the high rate of incomplete tests due to the need to have the test read between 48 and 72 hours of administration, has given way to IGRA testing.

TB IGRA Testing

IGRA tests are blood tests. There are two currently on the market, the QuantiFERON and the TB Spot. The TB Spot has slight preference as of this writing due to cost issues and savings that can be garnered as the laboratory who performs this test are willing to provide volume discounts. The advantage of this testing is that only one appointment is needed as there is no need to return as there is in skin testing.

In general, the procedure for these tests are specific by laboratory. Please refer to the individual laboratory instructions that are provided with the test collection kits.

Chest Radiography

A chest x-ray should be always be done within 72 hours of a positive TB test reading. A chest x-ray and sputum smear and culture should always be done within 72 hours of identification of symptoms of TB, such as:

- productive cough

- coughing up blood
- weight loss
- loss of appetite
- lethargy/weakness
- night sweats, or fever

Diagnosis of TB

Any individual with TB symptoms and/or chest x-ray indicative of TB will need further tests, such as sputum or other bacteriologic specimen for acid fast bacilli (AFB) smear and culture.

Initially, a series of three early morning sputum specimens should be collected on successive days and examined by smear and culture. Supervision should be used to ensure proper collection. (Cultures must be secretions brought up from the lungs (sputum), not from the nose or mouth (saliva). Patients may be told to inhale and exhale deeply three times and then inhale swiftly, cough deeply, and spit into the sputum container. Aerosol induction of sputum may be required. Sputum collections should be carried out in accordance with the necessary precautions as described previously in this document.

Until culture results return, the symptomatic patient is a suspect case. The only way to confirm the diagnosis of TB is by identifying *Mycobacterium tuberculosis* through culture. Drug susceptibility studies should be done on all initial specimens and on cultured bacilli from patients not responding to treatment.

Extra-Pulmonary TB

Diagnosis of extra-pulmonary TB can be difficult. Many sites other than the lungs can be affected, and symptoms will different for each site. When extra- pulmonary TB is suspected, other clinical specimens should be obtained: urine, pleural fluid, biopsy specimens, etc. Extra-pulmonary TB occurs more often in HIV-infected individuals than in persons without HIV infection.

Case Reporting

All suspected or diagnosed cases of tuberculosis should be reported to the health department according to state laws and regulations. Do not wait for results of sputum smears and cultures before reporting a suspect case of TB. The reporting of the TB case makes the resources of the health department available to assist in proper management of case and in the evaluation of contacts. In addition, the company shall maintain a reporting and record keeping system.

Additional Information

Please note the following four pages that contain a summarized general guideline with web link references plus a tuberculosis assessment form that may be used.

Tuberculosis Surveillance Testing Guideline

1. Core Curriculum on Tuberculosis: What the Clinician Should Know (Seventh Edition, 2021)
    a. Core Curriculum on Tuberculosis: What the Clinician Should Know (cdc.gov)
    b. DTBE | Interactive Core Curriculum on Tuberculosis | Main Menu (cdc.gov) (PowerPoint version that has not been updated since 2015)

2. Tuberculosis (TB) Symptom Assessment form

3. IGRA testing
    a. Complete testing per laboratory instructions
    b. A CXR cannot be substituted for a TST or IGRA unless otherwise described below.

4. For Health Care Workers/HealthCare students
    a. If no previous test or greater than 1 year since last test, complete IGRA

    b. Test results provided by another HCP may be accepted if
        i. Completed within the previous 12 months
        ii. Have person complete the Tuberculosis Symptom Assessment form.
            1. If any reports of TB symptoms on the form, proceed with IGRA.

5. Persons with a POSITIVE IGRA (initial finding) should be referred for further TB evaluation.
    a. Referral to their personal physician or Public Health

    b. CXR within 72 hrs. of a positive IGRA is desirable for timely diagnosis and exposure control of person with potential TB disease.

    c. Person must present documentation of a negative chest x-ray and physician note stating person is free of active TB disease.

6. IGRA (Interferon Gamma Release Assay)

    a. General information
        i. www.cdc.gov/mmwr/preview/mmwrhtml/rr5905a1.htm?s_cid=rr5905a1_e
        ii. Advantages
            1. Single appointment (no need to return)
            2. Persons who have had BCG vaccination

    b. QuantiFERON (QFT-GIT)
        i. Older IGRA
        ii. Instructions on collection and transport of specimen
        iii. https://www.questdiagnostics.com/home/physicians/testing-services/by-test-name/quantiferon/tb-plus-collection/#:~:text=%20QuantiFERON%20%C2%AE%20-TB%20Gold%20Plus%3Acollection%20instructions%20,Incubated%29.%20CPT%20coding%20is%20the%20sole...%20More%20

    c. T-Spot
        i. Newer IGRA
        ii. Cost is decreasing
        iii. Instructions on collection and transport of specimen
        iv. http://www.tspot.com/where-to-get-it/

7. History of BCG immunization
    a. Obtain history of immunization and if presence of TB symptoms

    b. Complete IGRA testing
        i. IGRAs are not affected by prior BCG vaccination and are not expected to give a false-positive result in people who have received BCG. www.cdc.gov/tb/topic/testing/default.htm

8. History of previous positive TST (documented or undocumented)
    a. Obtain history of testing, presence of TB symptoms

    b. Complete IGRA testing
        i. If positive IGRA then
            1. Refer to their personal physician or Public Health

2. Person must present documentation of a negative chest x-ray and physician note stating person is free of active TB disease.

ii. If negative IGRA then

1. Person must complete TB Symptom Assessment form

9. History of TB illness/disease
   a. Do not perform IGRA testing or CXR

   b. Person must provide documentation of previous assessment and completed treatment
      i. Person must complete TB Symptoms Questionnaire

   c. If person cannot provide documentation of previous assessment and completed treatment, then complete IGRA testing.

10. Consult Medical Director for guidance with any questions, how to manage equivocal IGRA results or any other unusual circumstances.

11. Additional Resource Websites:
    CDC Tuberculosis Homepage www.cdc.gov/tb/
    American Lung Association www.lung.org/lung-disease/tuberculosis/
    OSHA Tuberculosis www.osha.gov/SLTC/tuberculosis/

A person with latent TB infection (LTBI)	A person with TB disease
• Usually has a TB skin test or blood test result indicating TB infection	• Usually has a TB skin test or blood test result indicating TB infection
• Has a normal chest x-ray and a negative sputum test	• May have an abnormal chest x-ray, or positive sputum smear or culture
• Has TB bacteria in his/her body that are alive, but inactive	• Has active TB bacteria in his/her body

• Does not feel sick	• Usually feels sick and may have symptoms such as coughing, fever, and weight loss
• Cannot spread TB bacteria to others	• May spread TB bacteria to others
• Needs treatment for latent TB infection to prevent TB disease	• Needs treatment for TB disease

TUBERCULOSIS (TB) SYMPTOM ASSESSMENT

Name	DOB
Address	Phone
City/State/Zip	Company

PREVIOUS TB TESTING

Date of last TB Symptom Assessment:

____

Date of Positive TB skin test(s) and/or + IGRA tests:

____

Date of last Chest X-ray & results:

____

Date of completion, list of prior TB medications and prescribing provider:

____

Any known exposures to infectious TB? YES NO

If yes, explain:

TB Symptom Assessment

In the past 12 months have you had: (*check all that apply*)

- o Persistent or unexplained fever and/or chills
- o Night sweats (regardless of room temperature)
- o Persistent cough (more than 2-3 weeks) with or without phlegm
- o Cough up blood
- o Weakness or easily fatigued
- o Unexplained weight loss
- o Frequent colds or pneumonia
- o Any serious illness

I acknowledge that the above information is correct to the best of my knowledge.

Signature____

Date ____________________

Nurse Review____

Date ____________________

BLOODBORNE PATHOGENS
EXPOSURE CONTROL PROGRAM

For Compliance with OSHA Standard
Title 29, Code of Federal Regulations 1910.1030

Introduction

This Bloodborne Pathogens Exposure Control Program covers all employees who have occupational exposure to blood or other potentially infectious materials (OPIM). These employees will be identified on the Occupational Exposure Determination forms (See **Appendix A and B**). The listed employees will be trained in accordance with OSHA's 29 CFR 1910.1030 (g)(2) training requirements. All identified employees will adhere to the policies and procedures established in this Bloodborne Pathogens Exposure Control Program. This program will be made accessible, at all times, to employees as well as to OSHA and NIOSH representatives. Employees must be able to access a copy of this program at the workplace during the work shift. If the program is maintained solely on the computer, employees must be trained to operate the computer. A hard copy of the program must be provided within 15 working days of the employee's request.

POLICY STATEMENT

Knowledge of the health risks associated with potential occupational exposure to Bloodborne Pathogens and the communication of that knowledge to any employee who has risk of occupational exposure to Bloodborne Pathogens are considered high priorities and important objectives in overall worker safety and health. All employees who have a predetermined identified risk of occupational exposure to Bloodborne Pathogens, or who have received an occupational exposure to the blood of another person will be made aware of those risks.
This program has been developed to educate employees on the safe practices to eliminate or minimize occupational exposure to blood and certain other body fluids.

RESPONSIBILITY

The development and maintenance of this program is vested in the Safety Director and/or Occupational Health Nurse who will perform an annual review to assure compliance. They will also responsible for maintaining all records pertaining to the Exposure Control Program.
It is the responsibility of all employees to follow all policies and procedures contained within this program.

EXPOSURE DETERMINATION

Exposure determination must be based on the definition of occupational exposure without regard to personal protective clothing and equipment. All job classifications will be reviewed and those dealing with occupational exposure will be broken down into two groups and listed.

Job Classifications with Possible Occupational Exposure

The first group includes job classifications in which all employees have occupational exposure. These job classifications will be listed, although it is not necessary to list the specific work tasks of the people contained in this group. (See **Appendix A**)

The second group includes job classifications in which some of the employees have occupational exposure. For these job classifications, it will be necessary to list the specific tasks and procedures causing occupational exposure. (See **Appendix B**)

First Responders and Responsible Personnel

Responders and Responsible Personnel have been identified as having a potential occupational exposure to blood and/or Bloodborne Pathogens. Employees who volunteer for this assignment could be exposed to blood and Bloodborne Pathogens as a result of providing immediate first aid assistance on company property,or could be required to decontaminate or control contaminated equipment.

Any employee who has been identified as a First Responder will be required to sign a First Responder Information Form. This form will be maintained in the employee's personnel file. (See **Appendix C**)

Any employee who has been identified as a Responsible Person will be required to sign a Responsible Person Bloodborne Pathogen Exposure Control Statment. This form will be maintained in the employee's personnel file. (See **Appendix D**)

Preventative Measures

Universal Precautions

All employees will adhere to the Universal Precautions method. Universal Precautions are OSHA's required methods of control to protect employees from exposure to all human blood and other potentially infectious materials. The term "Universal Precautions" refers to a concept of bloodborne disease control which requires that all human blood and other potentially infectious materials be treated as known to be infectious for HIV, HBV (Hepetitis B Virus), HCV (Hepetitis C Virus) or other bloodborne pathogens.

Where differentiation of types of body fluids is difficult or impossible, all body fluids are to be considered potentially infectious.

Body Substance Isolation (BSI)

Body Substance Isolation is a control method that defines all body fluids and substance as infectious. BSI incorporates not only the fluids and materials covered by the standard but expands coverage to include all body substances. BSI is an acceptable alternative to Universal Precautions, provided facilities utilizing BSI adhere to all other provisions of the standard.

Engineering Controls

Engineering controls and work practice controls are to be the primary methods used to prevent occupational transmission of HBV and HIV.

Engineering Controls reduce employee exposure in the workplace by either removing or isolating the hazard or isolating the worker from exposure. Engineering controls must be examined and maintained or replaced on a scheduled basis.

All engineering controls that are in place must be in accordance with 29 CFR 1910.1030 (d).

Work Practice Controls

Engineering controls and work practice controls are to be the primary methods used to prevent occupational transmission of HBV and HIV.

General

Proper work practice controls change the manner in which a task is performed. Where the possibility of occupational exposure exists in the work place, the following controls should be utilized:

Restricting eating, drinking, smoking, applying cosmetics or lip balm, and handling contact lenses;

Prohibiting mouth pipetting (sucking up any biological fluids through a staw);

Preventing the storage of food and/or drink in refrigerators or other locations where blood or other potentially infectious materials are kept;

Providing and requiring the use of hand-washing facilities and/or equipment;

Routinely checking equipment and decontaminating it prior to servicing or shipping;

Washing hands when gloves are removed and as soon as possible after skin contact with blood or other potentially infectious materials occurs;

Recapping, removing or bending needles is prohibited unless the employer can demonstrate that no alternative is feasible or that such action is required by a specific medical procedure. When recapping, bending or removing contaminated needles is required by a medical procedure, this must be done by mechanical means, such as the use of forceps, or by a one-handed technique.

Shearing or breaking contaminated needles is not permitted.

The company will ensure that employees who handle or utilize knives or other sharp instruments have been trained in the safe and proper use of this equipment. Supervisors will ensure that box cutters or other sharp instruments are not left unattended in an open or unsheathed condition, where they can increase the potential for a puncture or laceration injury.

Hand Washing Facilities

Hand-washing facilities have been established throughout the facility. All persons who come in contact with the blood of another person or other potential infectious materials must wash their hands and any other skin with soap and water; if contact with eyes, mouth or nose, flush area with water immediately or as soon as possible following such contact. When hand-washing facilities are unavailable, employees will use antiseptic cleanser and paper towels or antiseptic towelettes. All employees must know where the hand-washing facilities and other hand-washing supplies are located.

SHARPS

Sharps containers must be made easily accessible to employees and located as close as feasible to the immediate area where sharps are used. Each sharps container must either be labeled with the universal biohazard symbol or word "biohazard" or be color-coded red. Sharps containers must also be closable, puncture resistant and leakproof on sides and bottom.

Contaminated needles and other sharps will not be bent, recapped, or removed unless it can be demonstrated that no alternative is feasible. Such bending, recapping or needle removal must be accomplished through the use of mechanical device or a one-handed technique.

Sharps containers will be maintained upright throughout use, replaced routinely, and not be allowed to overfill when removing sharps containers from the area of use, the containers shall be:

Closed immediately prior to removal or replacement to prevent spillage or protrusion of contents during handling, storage, transport, or shipping;

Placed in a secondary container if leakage is possible. The second container shall be: Closable; Constructed to contain all contents and prevent leakage during handling, storage, transport, or shipping; and Labeled or color-coded according to paragraph (g)(1)(i) of the standard.

Reusable containers shall not be opened, emptied, or cleaned manually or in any other manner which would expose employees to the risk of precutaneous injury.

Personal Protective Equipment

If occupational exposures remain after instituting engineering and work practice controls, Personal Protective Equipment (PPE) must be used.

Choosing and Using PPE

PPE is considered appropriate only if it does not permit blood or other potentially infectious materials to pass through or reach employees' work clothes, street clothes, undergarments, skin, eyes, mouth, or other mucous membranes under normal conditions of use and for the duration of the time which the PPE will be used. The protective equipment will be provided at no cost to the employee. A variety of sizes will be offered for the employee to select from.

Types of PPE include gloves, gowns, masks, mouthpieces and resuscitation bags. If the PPE is reusable, it must be repaired, replaced and/or cleaned when necessary. Cleaning procedures are outlined in the written schedule for cleaning. (See **Appendix E**)

Disposable PPE will not be reused. If circumstances require the use of this equipment, it will be properly disposed of after its use in the designated leak-proof container. The company will issue new PPE to the employee.

Employees utilizing PPE will remove the equipment prior to leaving the work area. Employees are not permitted to take their protective equipment home/

Spare PPE will be maintained. This equipment will be made available, as needed, to any person who renders first aid assistance.

First Responders and Responsible Personnel

First Responders and Responsible Personnel will have an Infection Protection Kit in their possession. Contents of an Infection Protection Kit should include the following items:

Antiseptic Towelettes

Rubber latex gloves

Face mask

Disposable body gown

Disposable shoe covers

Protective eye wear

Biohazard bag with secure tie

Area Control Biohazard warning tape and signs

First Responders certified in CPR will be provided with plastic mouth shields to protect a first responders' mouth area while performing Artificial Respiration or Cardiopulmonary Resuscitation (CPR).

All First Responders and Responsible Personnel will be required to use PPE at all times when performing first aid on another person or decontaminating suspected contaminated equipment, products, or materials. The circumstances under which any or all of this equipment will be used depend on the nature of the injury and the nature and extent of first aid assistance rendered. It will be the responsibility of each person rendering first aid assistance to use the appropriate degree of discretion and judgment necessary when deciding what type of PPE should be utilized for the given circumstances. However, in all cases, when rendering immediate first aid to a bleeding person, First Responders will be required to use all PPE in their assigned Infection Protection Kits. If the First Responder makes a judgment in a given circumstance, that the use of PPE will impede the delivery of first aid treatment or pose an increased hazard to the safety of the injured person or other employees, this judgment will be documented.

Housekeeping

The facility will be kept clean and sanitary at all times. Any surface that has been exposed to potentially infectious materials will be decontaminated. Types of disinfectant to use when decontaminating equipment or working surfaces which have come in contact with blood or OPIMs are included in **Appendix F**. A cleaning schedule has been developed that includes appropriate methods of decontamination and tasks or procedures to be performed (See **Appendix E**).

The following housekeeping procedures will be followed:

Clean and decontaminate all equipment and environmental and work surfaces that have been contaminated with blood or other potentially infectious materials.

Decontaminate work surfaces with an appropriate disinfectant after completion of procedures, immediately when overtly contaminated, after any spill of blood or other potentially infectious materials, and at the end of the work shift when surfaces have become contaminated since the last cleaning.

Remove and replace protective coverings, such as plastic wrap and aluminum foil, when contaminated.

Inspect and decontaminate, on a regular basis, reusable receptacles, such as bins, pails, and cans, that have a potential for becoming contaminated. When contamination is visible, clean and decontaminate receptacles immediately or as soon as feasible.

Always use mechanical means, such as tongs, forceps, or a brush and a dust pan to pick up contaminated broken glassware; never pick up with hands even if gloves are worn.

Store or process reusable sharps in a way that ensures safe handling.

Place other regulated waste in closable and labeled or color coded containers. When storing, handling, transporting or shipping, place other regulated waste in containers that are constructed to prevent leakage.

When discarding contaminated sharps, place them in containers that are closable, puncture-resistant, appropriately labeled or color-coded, and leakproof on the sides and bottom.

Ensure that sharps containers are easily accessible to personnel and located as close as is feasible to the immediate area where sharps are used or are reasonably anticipated to be found. Sharps containers also must be kept upright throughout use, replaced routinely, closed when moved, and not allowed to overfill.

Never manually open, empty, or clean reusable contaminated sharps disposal containers.

Discard all regulated waste according to federal, state, and local regulations.

Handle contaminated laundry as little as possible and with minimum agitation.

Use appropriate personal protective equipment when handling contaminated laundry.

Place wet contaminated laundry in leak-proof, labeled or color-coded containers before transporting.

Bag contaminated laundry at its location of use.

Never sort or rinse contaminated laundry in areas of its use.

Labeling

The company will ensure that warning labels, including the orange or orange-red biohazard symbol are affixed to containers of regulated waste, refrigerators and freezers and other containers which are used to store or transport blood or other potentially infectious materials. Red bags or containers may be used as a substitute for biohazard labels

Labeling is not required for:

Containers of blood, blood components, and blood products bearing an FDA required label that have been released for transfusion or other clinical uses.

Individual containers of blood or OPIM that are placed in secondary labeled containers during storage, transport, shipment, or disposal.

Specimen containers, if the facility uses Universal Precautions when handling all specimens, the containers are recognizable as containing specimens, and the containers remain within the facility.

Laundry bags or containers, containing contaminated laundry, may be marked with an alternative label or color-coded provided the facility uses Universal Precautions for handling all soiled laundry and the alternative marking permits all employees to recognize the containers as requiring compliance with Universal Precautions. If contaminated laundry is sent off-site for cleaning to a facility which does not use Universal Precautions in the handling of all soiled laundry, it must be placed in a bag or container which is red in color or labeled with the biohazard label described above.

Regulated waste that has been decontaminated.

Contaminated Laundry

Contaminated laundry will be handled as little as possible. If it is necessary to handle contaminated laundry, it will be bagged or placed in a container at the location where it was used. Such laundry will not be sorted or rinsed in the area of use. Bag and containers must be labeled or color-coded with biohazard labels for recognition that the contents within them are hazardous. The appropriate PPE will be selected and used when employees come in contact with contaminated laundry.

Laundries must have sharps containers easily accessible due to the risk of needles being mixed with laundry.

VACCINATIONS

The Hepatitis B vaccination is a noninfectious, yeast-based vaccine given in three injections in the arm. It is prepared from recombinant yeast cultures, rather than human blood or plasma. Therefore, there is no risk of contamination from other Bloodborne Pathogens, nor is there any chance of developing the Hepatitis B virus from the vaccine.

Employees

Hepatitis B vaccinations will be made available to all employees who have occupational exposure to blood within 10 working days of assignment, at no cost to the employee, at a reasonable time and place, under the supervision of a licensed physician/licensed healthcare professional, and according to the latest recommendations of the U.S. Public Health Service. The company will make all the necessary arrangements for the employee to obtain the pre-vaccination screening and vaccination. The Hepatitis B vaccination, post-exposure evaluation and follow-up for employees will be provided at the expense of the company with no cost to the employee. The Hepatitis B vaccination does not have to be made available to employees who have previously received the vaccination serires, who are already immune as their antibody tests reveal, or who are prohibited from receiving the vaccine for medical reasons.

An employee may, at his/her discretion, decline to be prescreened for the presence of Hepatitis B virus antibodies, but still receive the Hepatitis B vaccination (prescreening may not be required as a condition of receiving the vaccine). Employees must sign a declination form (See **Appendix H**) if they choose not to be vaccinated, but may later opt to receive the vaccine at no cost to the employee. Emplooyes that consent to the Hepatitis B vaccination will sign an approval form (See **Appendix G**). Both Declination and Approval forms will be filed with the employee's other confidential medical records.

The Safety Director and/or Occupational Health Nurse will request a written report from the designated medical provider who provides a Hepatitis B vaccination to the employee. This written report will document that the employee has in fact received the vaccination. They will ensure that a copy of the medical provider's written report is given to the employee within (15) working days of receipt.

If the U.S. Public Health Service recommends a routine dose(s) of Hepatitis B vaccine at a future date, such booster dose(s) will be made available at no charge.

First Responders and Other Responsible Persons

All employees identified as First Responders or Responsible Persons, at their discretion, will be eligible to be prescreened for the presence of Hepatitis B virus antibodies and to receive a Hepatitis B Vaccine at no cost to the employee within ten (10) working days of their assignment as a First Responder or Responsible Person.

The company will make Hepatitis B prescreening services and Hepatitis B vaccinations available to any employee designated as a First Responder who initially declines to be prescreened and vaccinated, but who decides at a later date that they would like to receive the prescreening and vaccination.

Although pre-vaccination screening and the Hepatitis B vaccine are encouraged, employees who are designated as First Responders may decline both the pre-vaccination screening and a Hepatitis B vaccination. Employees who decline a Hepatitis B vaccination must sign a Hepatitis B Vaccination Declination Form. (See **Appendix H**)

EXPOSURE INCIDENTS

An exposure incident may occur if an employee, acting either in the role of a First Responder, Good Samaritan, or Responsible Person, comes into contact with the blood of another person or some other potentially infectious material. An example of an employee subject to an exposure incident would be a First Responder or Good Samaritan rendering first aid assistance to a person who is bleeding. Another example would be a person receiving a laceration injury by an item that had previously been contaminated by the blood of another person. These exposure incidents are serious. All incidents that could expose an employee to blood or Bloodborne Pathogens must be well documented.

Safety Representative's Responsibilities

When any exposure incident occurs, the Safety Director and/or Occupational Health Nurse will ensure that the area and/or equipment that has been contaminated by blood or other potentially infectious materials is secured from inadvertent exposure to others by placing warning tape and signs around the contaminated area. Signs will not be removed until the area is thoroughly cleaned and disinfected with disinfectant solution by a Responsible Person wearing appropriate Personal Protective Equipment.

When any employee is subject to an exposure incident, regardless of whether or not that employee is a designated First Responder, the Safety Director and/or Occupational Health Nurse will:

immediately refer that employee to the designated medical provider.

ensure that the employee subjected to the exposure incident receives a confidential medical evaluation and follow up.

provide the designated medical provider with a copy of the completed Blood and Fluid Exposure Report as soon as possible following an investigation of the exposure incident. This worksheet will allow the medical provider to more accurately assess the employee's potential for exposure and what follow-up care should be provided.

request the source individual voluntarily submit to serological blood test to screen for the presence of Hepatitis B (HBV), Hepatitis C (HCV) and human immunodeficiency (HIV) virus antibodies (See **Appendix J**). If the source individual agrees to be tested, the person should be directed to the designated medical provider.

request the source individual provide the medical provider for the employee subjected to the exposure incident the results of all blood tests conducted on the source individual. The results of these tests will help the medical provider to determine the extent of the follow-up care for the employee who has been subjected to the exposure incident.

if the source individual refuses to voluntarily submit to blood testing, advise the medical provider that the source individual refused to be tested, and document the source individual's refusal to give consent for testing on the Blood Testing Consent/Non-Consent Form (See **Appendix J**).

if the source individual declines a blood test to determine the presence of human immunodeficiency (HIV) virus antibodies, but does give consent for a blood test to determine the presence of Hepatitis B (HBV) and Hepatitis C (HCV) antibodies, the company will advise the medical provider to retain the source individual's blood sample for a period of ninety (90) days following the date the source individual's blood was drawn. The source individual may elect to have a blood test to detect HIV antibodies at a later date, in which case the medical provider can use the original sample provided by the source individual.

request that the medical provider send a written report to the company documenting that the employee subjected to the exposure incident was informed of the medical evaluation results and the need for any further follow up. The Safety Director and/or Occupational Health Nurse will ensure that a copy of the medical providers report is given to the employee subjected to the exposure incident within (15) days after receipt.

Blood and Body Fluid Exposure Report

The Safety Director and/or Occupational Health Nurse must document the exposure incident on the Blood and Body Fluid Exposure Report (See **Appendix I**). They will ensure that the following minimum elements are addressed when completing the Blood and Body Fluid Exposure Report:

Identification of the employee(s) subjected to the exposure incident.

Identification of the "source individual(s)."

Documentation of whether the source individuals voluntarily consented to blood testing to determine the presence of Hepatitis B (HBV), Hepatitis C (HCV) or human immunodeficiency virus (HIV) in the source individual's blood.

Documentation of the route(s) of exposure and circumstances under which exposure occurred.

Whether any PPE was utilized by the First Responder when rendering first aid assistance. If PPE was not utilized, the reasons why should be documented on the worksheet.

Post-Exposure Evaluation, Follow-Up and Laboratory Tests

All post-exposure evaluation and follow-up plus laboratory tests conducted must be available, in confidence, to each employee who has had an exposure incident. The evaluations and test must be conducted by an accredited laboratory and provided at no cost to the employee. Follow-up must include a confidential medical evaluation documenting the following information:

Circumstances of the exposure,

Identifying and testing the source individual, if feasible,

Testing the exposed employee's blood if he/she consents,

Post-exposure prophylaxis, and

Counseling and evaluation of reported illnesses.

A copy of the medical provider's report on the employee subjected to the exposure incident will be filed with the employee's other confidential medical records.

Post-Exposure Counseling

Post-exposure counseling will be made availabe to exposed employees regardless of the employee's decision to accept serological testing. The counseling should include the U. S. Public Health Service (USPHS) recommendations for transmission and prevention of HIV. These recommendations include: refraining from blood, semen, or organ donation; abstaining from sexual intercourse or using measures to prevent HIV transmission during sexual intercourse; and refraining from breast feeding infants during the follow-up period.

TRAINING

All employees with occupational exposure must receive initial and annual training. Part-time and temporary employees are also to be trained on company time.

Bloodborne Pathogen Exposure control training will be held within 90 days of the effective date of hire, initially upon assignment, and annually. Employees who have received appropriate training within the past year need only receive additional training in items not previously covered. This training will be conducted by a person who is knowledgeable about the subject matter being presented. A medical nurse from our Contracted Health Care Provider will be contacted to provide the training. At the minimum, the training provided to all employees will cover the following areas:

An explanation of the contents of the Bloodborne Pathogen standard;

Where a copy of the text of the regulatory standard and the explanation of its contents is located;

The modes by which Bloodborne disease is transmitted;

An explanation of the Exposure Control Program;

Recognition of exposure situations;

Engineering and work practice controls;

Signs/labels/color-coding;

Associate practices to prevent exposure and contamination;

How to use Personal Protective Equipment;

Information on the Hepatitis B (HBV) vaccine;

Responses to emergencies involving blood;

Post-exposure evaluation and follow-up program.

The location and use of hazardous waste disposal containers

All employees who receive this training must sign the Training Log (See **Appendix K**), which documents the training. This log will be filed with records of the regularly scheduled employee training meetings and must be retained by the company for a period of three (3) years from the training date.
The Safety Director will provide every First Responder and Responsible Person with a hard copy of the Bloodborne Pathogens Exposure Control Program. The First Responder Information form is used to document the First Responder's receipt of the Exposure Control Program, and the Responsible Person Bloodborne Pathogen Exposure Control Statement is used to document the Responsible Person's receipt of the Exposure Control Program.
The Safety Director will provide to any employee who so requests, a print copy of the Bloodborne Pathogen Exposure Control Program no later than fifteen (15) working days from the date of the employee's request.

RECORDKEEPING

Medical Records

The company under the direction of the Safety Director and/or Occupational Health Nurse is responsible for maintaining medical records as indicated below. These records will be kept separate from the employees' personnel file and under lock and key in the Health Services office. Medical records will be maintained in accordance with OSHA Standard 29 CFR 1910.1020. These records will be kept confidential, and must be maintained for at least the duration of employment plus 30 years. The records will include the following:

The name and social security number of the employee.

A copy of the employees HBV vaccination status, including the dates of vaccination.

A copy of the results of examinations, medical testing, and follow-up procedures.

A copy of the information provided to the healthcare professional, including a description of the employee's duties as they relate to the exposure incident, and documentation of the routes of exposure and circumstances of the exposure.

Upon request, medical records must be made available to the Director of the National Institute for Occupational Safety and Health (NIOSH) and the Assistant Secretary of Labor for Occupational Safety and Health. An employee's medical records can be obtained by that employee or anyone having that employee's written consent. Also, if the employer ceases to do business, medical records must be transferred to the successor employer. If there is no successor employer, the employer must notify the Director, NIOSH, U.S. Department of Health and Human Services, for specific directions regarding disposition of the records at least 3 months prior to intended disposal.

Training Records

Training records will be maintained and kept for three years from the date of training. The following information will be included with the documentation:

The dates of the training sessions;

An outline describing the material presented;

The names and qualifications of persons conducting the training;

The names and job titles of all persons attending the training sessions.

Upon request, training records must be made available to the Director of the National Institute for Occupational Safety and Health (NIOSH) and the Assistant Secretary of Labor for Occupational Safety and Health. Training records must be available to employees or employee representatives upon request. Also, if the employer ceases to do business, training records must be transferred to the successor employer. If there is no successor employer, the employer must notify the Director, NIOSH,

U.S. Department of Health and Human Services, for specific directions regarding disposition of the records at least 3 months prior to intended disposal.

OSHA 300 Log

All occupational bloodborne pathogens exposure incidents, (e.g., needlesticks, lacerations, splashes), must be recorded on the OSHA 300 log as an injury if the incident results in one of the following:

The incident is work-related and involves the loss of consciousness, a transfer to another job, or restriction of work or motion.

The incident results in a recommendation of medical treatment, (e.g., Hepatitis B immune globulin, Hepatitis B vaccine, or Zidovudine)

The incident results in a diagnosis of seroconversion. The serological status of the employee is not recorded on the OHSA Log. If a case of seroconversion is known, it is recorded on the log as an injury, (e.g., "needlestick"), rather than "seroconversion".

Written Program Review

This program must be: (1) reviewed and updated at least annually or whenever new tasks and procedures affect occupational exposure, (2) made accessible to employees (in accordance with Title 29 CFR Part 1910.1020(e). Access to Employee Exposure and Medical Records) and (3) made available to the Assistant Secretary for OSHA and the Director of the National Institute for Occupational Safety and Health (NIOSH) for examination and copying.

Definition

Approved Disinfectant- A commercially available disinfectant such as Betacide or Madacide.

Blood- Human blood, human blood components and products made from human blood.

Bloodborne Pathogens- Pathogenic microorganisms that are present in human blood and can cause disease in humans. These Pathogens include, but are not limited to, Hepatitis B virus (HBV) and human immunodeficiency virus (HIV).

Care Giver- Any person who renders immediate first aid assistance to a person who has been injured on company property, acting in the role of either a First Responder or a Good Samaritan.

Contaminated- The presence or the reasonably anticipated presence of blood or other potentially infectious materials on an item or surface.

Contaminated Laundry- Laundry which has been soiled with blood or other potentially infectious materials or may contain sharps.

Contaminated Sharps- Any contaminated object that can penetrate the skin including, but not limited to, needles, scalpels, broken glass, broken capillary tubes, and exposed ends of dental wires.

Decontamination- The use of physical or chemical means to remove, inactivate, or destroy bloodborne pathogens on a surface or item to the point where they are no longer capable of transmitting infectious particles and the surface or item is rendered safe for handling, use, or disposal.

Engineering Controls- Controls (e.g., sharps disposal containers, self-sheathing needles) that isolate or remove the bloodborne pathogens hazard from the workplace.

Exposure Incident- A specific eye, mouth, other mucous membrane, non-intact skin, or parenteral contact with blood or other potentially infectious materials that result from the performance of an employee's duties.

First Responder- Any employee who has received accredited training in first aid and/or cardiopulmonary resuscitation (CPR) and has been designated as a person responsible for rendering immediate first aid assistance to persons who require emergency assistance while on company property.

Good Samaritan- Any person who voluntarily, and of their own free will, renders immediate first aid assistance to a person who is injured while on company property without legal or moral responsibility to do so.

Hand-washing Facilities- A facility providing an adequate supply of running potable water, soap, and single use towels or hot air drying machines.

HBV- Hepatitis B virus

HCV- Hepatits C virus

HIV- Human Immunodeficiency Virus

Licensed Healthcare Professional- A person whose legally permitted scope of practice allows him or her to independently perform the activities required by Hepatitis B Vaccination and Post-exposure Evaluation and Follow-up.

Occupational Exposure- Reasonably anticipated skin, eye, mucous membrane, or parenteral contact with blood or other potentially infectious materials that may result from the performance of an employee's duties.

Other Potentially Infectious Materials (OPIM) means:

The following human body fluids: semen, vaginal secretions, cerebrospinal fluid, synovial fluid, pleural fluid, pericardial fluid, peritoneal fluid, amniotic fluid, saliva in dental procedures, any body fluid that is visibly contaminated with blood, and all body fluids in situations where it is difficult or impossible to differentiate between body fluids;

Any unfixed tissue or organ (other than intact skin) from a human (living or dead); and

HIV-containing cell or tissue cultures, organ cultures, and HIV- or HBV containing culture medium or other solutions; and blood, organs, or other tissues from experimental animals infected with HIV or HBV.

Parenteral- Piercing mucous membranes or the skin barrier through such events as needlesticks, human bites, cuts, and abrasions.

Personal Protective Equipment- Specialized clothing or equipment worn by an employee for protection against a hazard. General work clothes (e.g., uniforms, pants, shirts or blouses) not intended to function as protection against a hazard are not considered to be personal protective equipment.

Regulated Waste- Liquid or semi-liquid blood or other potentially infectious materials; contaminated items that would release blood or other potentially infectious materials in a liquid or semi-liquid state if compressed; items that are caked with dried blood or other potentially infectious materials and are capable of releasing these materials during handling; contaminated sharps; and pathological and microbiological wastes containing blood or other potentially infectious materials.

Responsible Person (Personnel)- Any person or persons trained in the control of disinfection procedures and disposal procedures of equipment, product or materials suspected to be contaminated with Bloodborne Pathogens.

Source Individual- Any individual, living or dead, whose blood or other potentially infectious materials may be a source of occupational exposure to the employee.

Sterilize- The use of a physical or chemical procedure to destroy all microbial life including highly resistant bacterial endospores.

Universal Precautions- An approach to infection control. According to the concept of Universal Precautions, all human blood and certain human body fluids are treated as if known to be infectious for HIV, HBV, and other bloodborne pathogens.

Work Practice Controls- Controls that reduce the likelihood of exposure by altering the manner in which a task is performed (e.g., prohibiting recapping of needles by a two-handed technique).

Appendix A Job Classifications in Which All Employees Have Occupational Exposure

Employee Name	Job Title

Appendix B Job Classification in Which Some of the Employees Have Occupational Exposure

Employee Name	Job Title	Specific Tasks and Procedures or Groups of Closely Related Task and Procedures in Which Occupational Exposure Occurs

Appendix C First Responder Information Form

Name:		SSN:	
Division/ Dept.:		Job Title:	

First Aid Certification

Expiration Date: ____________________

County/State of Issue: ____________________

Cardiopulmonary Resuscitation Certification

Certificate Number: ____________________

Expiration Date: ____________________

Agency Issuing Certificate: ____________________

Emergency Medical Technician Certification

Certification Number: ____________________

Certificate Date: ____________________

Expiration Date: ____________________

County/State of Issue:

As a volunteer First Responder, I understand that I may be exposed to blood or Bloodborne Pathogens during the course of providing immediate first aid assistance to others. I have received a copy of the Bloodborne Pathogen Exposure Control Program. I have had an opportunity to review the Exposure Control Program, and I am familiar with all provisions to reduce my risk of exposure to blood and Bloodborne Pathogens outlined in the Exposure Control Program.

I understand that my role as a First Responder is voluntary and that I will receive no monetary or other material compensation for my services as a First Responder. I understand that I may withdraw my consent to act as a designated First Responder at any time.

Signature:		Date:	

Appendix D Responsible Person's Bloodborne Pathogen Exposure Control Statement

As a designated Responsible Person, I understand that in the course of work I may be requested to decontaminate equipment or facilities, or control materials contaminated with blood or other body fluids which could carry Pathogens capable of causing diseases including, but not limited to, Hepatitis B Virus (HBV), Hepatitis C Virus (HCV) and human immunodeficiency virus (HIV). I have received training on control measures and have received and read the company Exposure Control Program.

I will do anything conceivably possible to protect myself and my fellow workers from potential exposures to Bloodborne Pathogens.

Signature:		**Date:**	

Appendix E Cleaning Schedule Including Appropriate Methods of Decontamination and Tasks or Procedures to Be Performed

(please insert cleaning schedule and methods here)

Appendix F OSHA's Suggested Types of Disinfectants to Use When Decontaminating Equipment or Working Surface Which Have Come in Contact with Blood or OPIM

EPA registered tuberculocidal disinfectants are appropriate for the cleaning of blood or OPIM. A solution of 5.25 percent sodium hypochlorite, (household bleach), diluted between 1:10 and 1:100 with water, is also acceptable for cleaning contaminated surfaces. Quaternary ammonium products are appropriate for use in general housekeeping procedures that do not involve the cleanup of contaminated items or surfaces. The particular disinfectant used, as well as the frequency with which it is used, will depend upon the circumstances in which a given housekeeping task occurs (i.e., location within the facility, type of surface to be cleaned, type of soil present, and tasks and procedures being performed).

Appendix G Hepatitis B Vaccine Approval Form

I, ______________________________, wish to receive a series of three vaccinations for Hepatitis B. The vaccine is prepared from yeast cultures and is free from association with human blood. The series will be provided to me at no cost by my employer, (______________________________). I understand I must remain in the first aid room for observation for 15 minutes following the injection.

Employee Signature:		**Date:**	

Please Complete:

Known Medical Allergies: ______________________________

____

Any known medical conditions: ______________________________

(If the possibility of pregnancy exists, you must first discuss risks with your physician) ______________________________

Injection #1 given:

(Date)	(Nurse's Signature)

(Lot #)	(Agent)	(Dose)	(Route)	(Site)

Injection #2 given:

(Date)	(Nurse's Signature)

(Lot #)	(Agent)	(Dose)	(Route)	(Site)

Injection #3 given:

(Date) (Nurse's Signature)

(Lot #)	(Agent)	(Dose)	(Route)	(Site)

Appendix H Hepatitis B Vaccine Declination Form

I understand that due to my occupational exposure to blood or other potentially infectious materials, I may be at risk of acquiring Hepatitis B virus (HBV) infection. I have been given the opportunity to be vaccinated with Hepatitis B vaccine at no charge to myself.

However, I decline Hepatitis B vaccination at this time. I understand that by declining this vaccine, I continue to be at risk of acquiring Hepatitis B, a serious disease. If, in the future I continue to have occupational exposure to blood or other potentially infectious materials and I want to be vaccinated with Hepatitis B vaccine, I can receive the vaccination series at no charge to me.

Name of Employee (print)	Employee Number
Signature of Employee	Date Signed

Appendix I **Blood and Body Fluid Exposure Report**

Employee Name:		**Date of Birth:**	

SSN:		**Employee #:**		**Dept. #:**	
Job Title:					

Hepatitis B Vaccination status:	☐ Series complete		☐ In process		☐ Denied
Injection Dates:	# 1	# 2		# 3	
Date of Exposure:					
Date Exposure Reported:					

Time of Exposure (Approximate, if unknown):		
Responsible Person:	☐ Yes	☐ No
Good Samaritan:	☐ Yes	☐ No
Description of the Incident: (Include causes, where and how it occurred, and body parts involved.)		
Body Fluids Involved:	☐ Yes	☐ No
Exposure was to:	☐ Non-Intact Skin	☐ Intact Skin
Exposure source known?	☐ Yes	☐ No
Consent obtained for HIV/HBV testing? (If yes, nameless copy of lab results attached to this form.)	☐ Yes	☐ No
Indicate type of Personal Protective Equipment (PPE) used for this procedure:	☐ Glove	☐ Goggles

	☐ Mask ☐ Gown		☐ None ☐ Other	
Was the PPE available for your use: If NO, indicate why not:	☐ Yes ☐ Don't know		☐ No ☐ N/A	
Referred to:		Phone:		
Additional Comments:				
Completed?	☐ Injury/Illness Report ☐ OSHA 300 Log ☐ First Report of Injury (Workers' Compensation Claim Form)			

Name of Preparer (print) | Title of Preparer | Date Form Completed

Appendix J Blood Testing Consent/Non-Consent Form

Date of Exposure Incident:	
Hepatitis B Vaccination Status	☐ **Series complete** ☐ **In process** ☐ **Has not been vaccinated**

I, ________________________________, consent to being tested, as indicated below, for HIV and/or HBV and HCV. I understand that the results of this testing will be kept confidential and will be used to determine appropriate treatment for the individual exposed to my blood or body fluid. The test will be paid for by (____).

Consent is given to be tested for:		
HIV (Human Immunodeficiency Virus)	☐ **Yes**	☐ **No**
HBV (Hepatitis B Virus)	☐ **Yes**	☐ **No**
HCV (Hepatitis C Virus)	☐ **Yes**	☐ **No**

(Employee Name)	**(Employee #)**	**(Date)**

I, ________________________________, do not consent to any blood testing. The circumstances for the request to do so have been explained to me and I have no further questions or comments that need to be addressed as I make this decision. I understand that this denial will be kept confidential.

(Employee Name	**(Employee #)**	**(Date)**

Appendix K Bloodborne Pathogen Training Certificate

I have received Bloodborne Pathogen Training as described in Section 8.0 of this Bloodborne Pathogen Policy. The training was conducted on ____________________ (date).

(Employee Signature)

(Social Security Number)

(Work Area/Department)

I certify that the above-named employee has been provided with Bloodborne Pathogen Training on ____________________ (date).

(Instructor's Signature)

Workplace Violence Policy

PURPOSE: To ensure the highest standard of health and safety for all employees and mandates a "zero tolerance for violence".

SCOPE: Covers all employees who are employed (full-time, part-time, contractors).

METHODS OF COMPLIANCE: Requires prompt and accurate reporting of **all** violent incidents. Mandates that all reports be investigated, and information be kept confidential, except where there is a need to know in order to effectuate a solution to the problem. Establishes criteria for employee counseling in the event a major violent incident occurs. Prohibits discrimination against victims of work place violence. The plan limits access to all property to those with a legitimate business interest and outlines procedures for allowing entry. Prohibits the carrying of any type of weapon onto company property. Requires that all employees receive training in the definition of workplace violence, a full explanation and full description of the organizations program, how to report all violent incidents, including threats and verbal abuse, recognizing and responding to workplace security hazards, identifying potential workplace security hazards, , methods for diffusing hostile or threatening situations, procedures for summoning assistance in case of an emergency or hostage situation, and post-incident procedures, including medical follow-up and the availability of counseling and referral.

RESOURCE LIST

Center for Disease Control www.cdc.gov

Siouxland District Health Department www.siouxlanddistricthealth.org

Iowa Department of Public Health www.idph.state.ia.us

ODG Treatment in Workers Compensation, 2021

ACOEM Practice Guidelines, 2021

Encyclopedia of Occupational Health & Safety, Online Edition, 2012

Manual of Emergency Medicine, 6th edition, Braen, Lippincott, 2011

Bedside Diagnostic Examination, DeGowin & DeGowin, 1981

Ophthalmology Principles and Concepts, 8th edition, Newell, Mosby, 1996

Siouxland Council on Sexual Assault and Domestic Violence

Sheehy's Manual of Emergency Care, 7th edition, Hammond and Zimmerman, ENA, 2012

Neuromotor Examination of the Limbs: A Photographic Atlas, Williams and Wilkins, 1980

Anatomy, Ciba-Geigy, 2021

Baum's Textbook of Pulmonary Diseases, Crapo et al. Lippincott, 2003

Physician's Desk Reference 2021

Ergonomic Program Management Guidelines for Meatpacking Plants, OSHA, 1990

Fundamentals of Occupational Safety and Health, 7th edition, Friend and Kohn, Littleton, 2018

Occupational Health Nursing Guidelines for Primary Clinical Conditions, Rogers et al., 2017

EEOC Technical Compliance Manual, Americans With Disabilities Act

Core Curriculum for Occupational and Environmental Health Nursing, Third Edition, AAOHN, Saunders, 2005

Instant Medical Surveillance, Mitchell, OEM Press, 2007

Medtronic, Inc. Implementation Guidelines for AEDs

UpToDate www.uptodate.com

www.ingramcontent.com/pod-product-compliance
Lightning Source LLC
LaVergne TN
LVHW070951210926
848482LV00002B/178
* 9 7 8 0 9 9 6 1 2 4 4 2 3 *